SURGEON'S GUIDE TO STAGING, GRADING & CLASSIFICATIONS

SURGEON'S GUIDE TO STAGING, GRADING & CLASSIFICATIONS

Lisa R. David, M.D.
Assistant Professor of Plastic & Reconstructive Surgery
Wake Forest University School of Medicine
Winston-Salem, North Carolina

Andrew M. Schneider, M.D.
Clinical Assistant Professor of Plastic & Reconstructive Surgery
Wake Forest University School of Medicine
Winston-Salem, North Carolina

Forsyth Plastic Surgical Associates
Winston-Salem, North Carolina

W.B. SAUNDERS COMPANY
A Harcourt Health Sciences Company

PHILADELPHIA   LONDON   NEW YORK   ST. LOUIS   SYDNEY   TORONTO

W.B. SAUNDERS COMPANY
A Harcourt Health Sciences Company

The Curtis Center
Independence Square West
Philadelphia, Pennsylvania 19106

Library of Congress Cataloging-in-Publication Data

David, Lisa R.
  Surgeon's guide to staging, grading & classifications / Lisa R. David, Andrew M.
Schneider.—1st ed.

    p. ; cm.

  ISBN 0–7216–8807–1

    1. Surgery—Classification—Handbooks, manuals, etc. I. Title: Surgeon's guide to
staging, grading, and classifications. II. Schneider, Andrew M. III. Title.
    [DNLM: 1. Classification—methods—Handbooks. 2. Surgical Procedures,
Operative—classification—Handbooks. 3. Severity of Illness Index—Handbooks.
  4. Trauma Severity Indices—Handbooks. WO 39 D249s 2001]

RD31.5 .D395 2001
617′.001′2—dc21

00-038807

Acquisitions Editor: Lisette Bralow
Project Manager: Edna Dick
Production Manager: Natalie Ware
Illustration Specialist: Lisa Lambert
Book Designer: Sasha O'Malley

SURGEON'S GUIDE TO STAGING, GRADING & CLASSIFICATIONS   ISBN 0-7216-8807-1

Printed in the United States of America

Last digit is the print number: 9   8   7   6   5   4   3   2   1

This book is dedicated to my wife Nancy, who I would classify as wonderful, and to my grade "A" children Bradley and Joel.

ANDREW M. SCHNEIDER

This book is dedicated to my husband Patrick, who is in a class all his own.

LISA R. DAVID

We would also like to dedicate this book to Dr. Tim Pennell, a gifted surgeon, educator, and administrator, who has inspired more than a generation of surgical residents at Wake Forest University.

FOREWORD

This text by Drs. Schneider and David fulfills an important need in the assessment, management, and long-term care of our patients. Medicine has become an increasingly complex endeavor, with an endless array of specialists ministering to the patient. At the same time these specialists are attempting to communicate with one another in a meaningful manner. Simultaneously, public health authorities, the "health care systems," and government agencies are seeking to monitor the effectiveness of treatment and cost-effectiveness of that treatment.

There are innumerable classifications of disease processes, many of which are not immediately available to those of us who practice clinical medicine. Many classifications have become so subdivided that they become difficult to remember but remain crucial for patient care. By having available the commonly defined systems of classification for most of the surgical diseases, the authors have allowed the patient, the treating physician, the consultant, the public health specialist, and the other medical care providers to function on the same "playing field." With appropriate classification of a patient's disease process, errors in treatment and follow-up can be avoided.

As a mentor for both these authors in the specialty of Plastic and Reconstructive Surgery, I am especially gratified that they have undertaken the important and difficult task of organizing this body of diverse material. Their holistic approach to the patient and his or her disease is particularly gratifying in this world of the superspecialized physician. This book will help all of us in medicine and surgery. More importantly, however, it will help our patients.

LOUIS C. ARGENTA, M.D.
Professor and Chairman
Department of Plastic & Reconstructive Surgery
Wake Forest University School of Medicine
Winston-Salem, North Carolina

PREFACE

"This patient has a Grade III splenic laceration," says the chief resident as she looks at the CT scan. Everyone nods in agreement.

But does everyone involved in the care of the patient really know what a Grade III splenic laceration is? We would like to think so, but the reality is that there are so many classification and grading schemes in 21st century medicine and surgery that no one person can remember them all (although some of our surgical mentors might have disagreed). It is for that reason we have assembled this work.

It is our hope that having a single, concise manual of staging and grading will lead to more accurate communication among surgeons, internists, and other medical professionals. We have put together the classification systems that are most likely used on a daily basis. A "complete" list would have required multiple volumes and perhaps have been unusable. There are certain to be systems of staging and grading that are important, widely known, and unfortunately not included. Let us know what you think is missing and we can attempt to include it in future editions. We sincerely hope that this work will be a useful part of any medical library and will be one of those rare texts that is frequently pulled off the shelf during the course of a day's work.

Please contact us at surgstag@wfubmc.edu regarding staging and grading systems that you think should be added to future editions of the text. We sincerely want your feedback.

LISA R. DAVID
ANDREW M. SCHNEIDER

ACKNOWLEDGMENTS

This book would not have been possible without our editorial assistant, Richard Worf. Rich undertook the often frustrating process of securing permissions from a multitude of different sources so that we might print previously published material. In fact, most of the data in this work have been published before, and therefore we had to contact many different sources. Sometimes the process was straightforward, but often it was confusing and time-consuming. Thanks, Rich, and good luck at Harvard.

We also want to thank Lisette Bralow at W.B. Saunders. Lisette gave us the chance to put this "non-book" together. "Hasn't it been done before?" she asked during our first phone call. Believe it or not, we said, there has never been a comprehensive compendium of grading and staging systems from the many surgical specialties. Thanks, Lisette, for supporting our project.

Lisa R. David
Andrew M. Schneider

CONTENTS

CHAPTER THREE
Cardiothoracic Surgery

CHAPTER FOUR
Trauma and Burn Surgery

CHAPTER FIVE
Pediatric Surgery

CHAPTER SIX
Plastic Surgery

CHAPTER SEVEN
Orthopedic and Hand Surgery

CHAPTER EIGHT
Head and Neck Surgery

CHAPTER NINE
Transplant Surgery

CHAPTER TEN
Oncology

CHAPTER ELEVEN
Urology

CHAPTER TWELVE
Neurosurgery

CHAPTER THIRTEEN
Anesthesia

Index

CHAPTER ONE

General Surgery

MODIFIED ALONSO-LEJ CLASSIFICATION OF BILE DUCT CYSTS

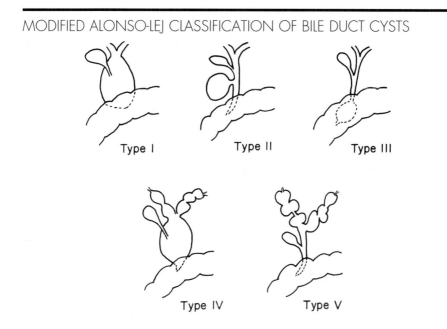

Type I Type II Type III

Type IV Type V

TYPE   DESCRIPTION

TYPE	DESCRIPTION
I	Fusiform or saccular dilatation of the common bile duct
II	Biliary diverticulum off a normal common bile duct
III	Cystic dilation of the bile duct in the intraduodenal region (choledochocele)
IV	Combined extra- and intrahepatic duct cystic dilatations
V	Biliary cystic dilatation limited to the intrahepatic region (Caroli's disease)

All choledochal cysts are premalignant lesions; if the cyst can be resected and the bile duct reconstructed surgically, it should be done once the diagnosis is made. Unfortunately, types IV and V cannot be completely resected and thus treatment is oriented around symptomatology.

From Alonso-Lej F, Rever WB, Pessagrio DJ: Congenital choledochal cysts, with a report of 2 and an analysis of 94 cases. Surg Gynecol Obstet 1959; 108:1–30.

CLASSIFICATION OF MESENTERIC CYSTS

TYPE 1 (EMBRYONIC AND DEVELOPMENTAL)
A. Enteric
B. Urogenital
C. Dermoid
D. Embryonic defects of the lymphatics
TYPE II (TRAUMATIC OR ACQUIRED)
A. Postoperative or penetrating trauma
B. Pseudocysts
C. Secondary to lymphatic rupture
TYPE III (NEOPLASTIC CYSTS)
A. Benign
B. Malignant
    1. Primary cystic malignancy
    2. Secondary cystic degeneration of solid malignancy
TYPE IV (INFECTIVE AND DEGENERATIVE CYSTS)
A. Mycotic cysts
B. Parasitic cysts
C. Tuberculous cysts

From Beahrs OH, Judd ES, Dockerty MB: Chylous cyst of the abdomen. Surg Clin North Am 1950; 30:1081.

RANSON'S EARLY PROGNOSTIC SIGNS OF ACUTE PANCREATITIS

I. Characteristics at time of admission
  a. Age over 55 years
  b. White blood cell count greater than 16,000 cells/mm^3
  c. Blood glucose > 200 mg/dL
  d. Serum lactate dehydrogenase > 350 IU/L
  e. SGOT > 250 U/dL
II. Characteristics after initial 48 hours
  a. Hematocrit fall > 10 percentage points
  b. BUN elevation > 5 mg/dL
  c. Serum calcium fall to < 8 mg/dL
  d. Arterial Po_2 < 60 torr
  e. Base deficit > 4 mEq/L
  f. Estimated fluid sequestration greater than 6 L
Patients with three or four prognostic signs have a mortality that approximates 15% with the majority requiring intensive care unit support.

BUN, blood urea nitrogen; SGOT, serum glutamic-oxalo-acetic transaminase.

From Ranson JHC, Rifkind KM, Roses DF, et al.: Prognostic signs and the role of operative management in acute pancreatitis. Surg Gynecol Obstet 1974; 139:69.

CLASSIFICATION OF FUNCTIONAL PANCREATIC ENDOCRINE TUMORS

TUMOR	HORMONE	CELL TYPE	SYNDROME	MALIGNANCY RATE	EXTRAPANCREATIC LOCATION
Insulinoma	Insulin	Beta cell	Hypoglycemia	<15%	Rare
Gastrinoma (Zollinger-Ellison syndrome)	Gastrin	Non-beta	Peptic ulcer Diarrhea	50%	Frequent
VIPoma (Verner-Morrison syndrome)	Vasoactive intestinal polypeptide	Non-beta	Diarrhea Hypokalemia Achlorhydria	Majority	Occasional
Glucagonoma	Glucagon	Alpha cell	Hyperglycemia Dermatitis	Majority	Rare
Somatostatinoma	Somatostatin	Delta cell	Hyperglycemia Steatorrhea	Majority	Rare

From Sabiston DC (ed): Textbook of Surgery, 14th ed. Philadelphia: W.B. Saunders, 1991: 1098.

CLASSIFICATION OF MALABSORPTION SYNDROMES

TYPE 1 (Intraluminal factors)

A. Decrease in effective length
  1. Resection of stomach or small bowel
  2. Intestinal fistulization
  3. Hypermotility
B. Decreased digestive activity
  1. Pancreatic
    a. Pancreatitis
    b. Carcinoma of the pancreas
    c. Pancreatectomy
    d. Cystic fibrosis
    e. Pancreatic duct lithiasis with obstruction
    f. Pancreaticocutaneous fistula
  2. Bile
    a. Hepatitis
    b. Cirrhosis
    c. T-tube drainage
    d. Biliary obstruction
    e. Inadequate resorption of bile salts
    f. Congenital absence of bile salts
C. Changes in microorganism population
  1. Blind loop
  2. Small intestinal diverticula
  3. Intestinal stasis
    a. Visceral neuropathy
    b. Primary neurologic diseases
    c. Scleroderma
    d. Partial obstruction
  4. Oral antibiotics
  5. Giardiasis
  6. Acute infectious diarrhea
  7. Gastric achlorhydria

TYPE II (Changes in the intestinal wall)

A. Mucosal epithelial cell
  1. Celiac disease of childhood
  2. Gluten-induced enteropathy
  3. Tropical sprue
  4. Disaccharidase deficiency
  5. Radiation enteritis
  6. Drug induced
  7. Triglyceride enzyme deficiency
B. Ground substance
  1. Lymphoma, leukemia
  2. Whipple's disease
  3. Regional enteritis
  4. Systemic mast cell disease
  5. Amyloidosis

CLASSIFICATION OF MALABSORPTION SYNDROMES *Continued*

      6. Tuberculosis

      7. Sarcoma, carcinoma

TYPE III (Abnormalities in blood or lymphatic channels)

A. Blood

    1. Arterial or venous insufficiency

    2. Congestive heart failure

    3. Vasculitis

B. Lymphatics

    1. Intestinal lymphangiectasis

    2. Lymphatic obstruction

TYPE IV (Indeterminate)

A. Zollinger-Ellison syndrome

B. Malignant carcinoid

C. Abetalipoproteinemia

D. Protein-losing enteropathy

E. Pernicious anemia

F. Hyperthyroidism

G. Hypoparathyroidism

H. Pneumatosis cystoides intestinalis

 I. Hemochromatosis

J. Kwashiorkor

K. Hypogammaglobulinemia

L. Adrenal-pituitary insufficiency

M. Tabes mesenterica

From Johnson CF: Malabsorption syndromes: Clinical and theoretical consideration.
Postgrad Med J 1965; 37:667.

CLASSIFICATION OF SURGICAL INFECTIONS

TYPE I—RELATIVE TO FINAL OUTCOME

A. Self-limiting

B. Serious infections requiring treatment

C. Fulminating infections

TYPE II—RELATIVE TO TIME OF ONSET

A. Anteoperative surgical infections

    1. Time and portal of entry are known

    2. Time and portal of entry are unknown

B. Operative surgical infections

    1. Preventable

    2. Nonpreventable

C. Postoperative surgical infections

    1. Wound infection

    2. Respiratory infection

    3. Urinary tract infection

From Meleney FL: Treatise on Surgical Infections. New York: Oxford University Press, 1948.

CLASSIFICATION OF SURGICAL WOUNDS ACCORDING TO RISK OF INFECTION

TYPE	DEFINITION	UNACCEPTABLE INFECTION RATE AT 30 DAYS
Clean	Nontraumatic No break in technique Respiratory, GI, GU tract not entered	>1.5%
Clean-contaminated	GI or respiratory tract entered without significant spillage Oropharynx, vagina, or noninfected GU or biliary tract entered Minor break in technique	>3%
Contaminated	Major break in technique Traumatic wound Gross spillage from GI tract Entrance into GU or biliary tract in presence of infected urine or bile	>5%

Infection is defined as the discharge of any purulent material.

GI, gastrointestinal; GU, genitourinary.

From Sabiston DC (ed): Textbook of Surgery, 14th ed. Philadelphia: W.B. Saunders, 1991:222.

CLASSIFICATION OF CIRRHOSIS

MORPHOLOGIC SCHEME
A. Macronodular
B. Micronodular
C. Mixed

HISTOLOGIC SCHEME
A. Portal
B. Postnecrotic
C. Posthepatic
D. Primary obstructive
E. Venoocclusive

ETIOLOGIC SCHEME
A. Alcohol
B. Viral hepatitis
C. Biliary obstruction
D. Venoocclusive
E. Hemochromatosis
F. Wilson's disease
G. Autoimmune
H. Syphilis
I. Drugs and toxins
J. Alpha-1-Antitrypsin deficiency
K. Cystic fibrosis
L. Glycogen storage
M. Sarcoidosis
N. Copper
O. Small bowel bypass
P. Idiopathic

There are many causes of cirrhosis, but often the clinical end result is the same—progressive liver failure leading to no hepatic function.

From Conn HO, Atterbury CE: Cirrhosis. In Schiff L, Schiff ER (eds): Diseases of the Liver, 6th ed. Philadelphia: J.B. Lippincott, 1987:726.

PATHOLOGIC CLASSIFICATION OF ACUTE HEPATIC FAILURE

CHARACTERISTIC	TYPE I	TYPE II
Serum aminotransferase	Markedly elevated	Elevated
Hepatic histology	Patchy areas of confluent necrosis	Microvesicular fatty infiltration
Causes	Hepatitis viruses Halothane Acetaminophen Isoniazid	Pregnancy Tetracycline

From Zakim D, Boyer TD: Hepatology: A Textbook of Liver Disease. Philadelphia: W.B. Saunders, 1982:417.

CHILD'S CRITERIA FOR HEPATIC FUNCTIONAL RESERVE

CRITERIA	A (MINIMAL)	B (MODERATE)	C (ADVANCED)
Serum bilirubin	<2.0 mg/dL	2–3.0 mg/dL	>3.0 mg/dL
Serum albumin	>3.5 g/dL	3–3.5 g/dL	<3.0 g/dL
Ascites	None	Easily controlled	Poorly controlled
Neurologic disorders	None	Minimal	Advanced
Nutrition	Excellent	Good	Poor, wasting

In most clinical series, operative mortality for Child's Class A, B, and C is 0% to 5%, 10% to 15%, and > 25%, respectively.

From Boyer TD: Portal hypertension and its complications: Bleeding esophageal varices, ascites, and spontaneous bacterial peritonitis. In Zakim D, Boyer TD (eds): Hepatology: A Textbook of Liver Disease. Philadelphia: W.B. Saunders, 1982:464–499.

CLASSIFICATION OF RETROPERITONEAL FIBROSIS

TYPE	ETIOLOGY
I	Idiopathic
II	Ergot derivatives
III	Malignancies
IV	Inflammatory disease A. Systemic inflammatory disease B. Inflammatory abdominal aortic aneurysm C. Bacterial
V	Other

From Koep L, Zuidema GD: The clinical significance of retroperitoneal fibrosis. Surgery 1977; 81:250.

CLASSIFICATION OF HIATAL HERNIAS

TYPE	DESCRIPTION
I (Sliding)	Result of an extension of the endoabdominal fascia through the hiatus, allowing the gastroesophageal junction to be displaced upward into the chest. There is no true peritoneal sac. Most common type.
II (Paraesophageal)	A true herniation of the stomach into a peritoneal sac in the mediastinum. Gastroesophageal junction in normal position.

ESOPHAGEAL MUCOSA

ESOPHAGEAL MUSCLE

SQUAMO COLUMNAR JUNCTION

PHRENO-ESOPHAGEAL MEMBRANE

STOMACH

ENDOTHORACIC FASCIA

DIAPHRAGM

ENDOABDOMINAL FASCIA

PERITONEUM

TYPE I
HIATAL HERNIA

ESOPHAGEAL MUSCLE

STOMACH

PHRENO-ESOPHAGEAL MEMBRANE

SQUAMO COLUMNAR JUNCTION

PERITONEAL SAC

ENDOTHORACIC FASCIA

DIAPHRAGM

ENDOABDOMINAL FASCIA

PERITONEUM

TYPE II
HIATAL HERNIA

The distinction is important because the management is different. The Type I hernia is usually managed medically, whereas the Type II hernia is considered a surgical emergency.

From Sabiston DC (ed): Textbook of Surgery, 14th ed. Philadelphia: W.B. Saunders, 1991: 706–707.

ENDOSCOPIC GRADES OF ESOPHAGITIS
SKINNER AND BELSEY CLASSIFICATION

GRADE	DESCRIPTION
I	Distal esophageal mucosal erythema
II	Mucosal erythema with superficial ulceration, typically linear and vertical with an overlying fibrinous membranous exudate that is easily wiped away, leaving a bleeding surface
III	Mucosal erythema with superficial ulceration and associated submucosal fibrosis on biopsy with a dilatable early stricture
IV	Extensive ulceration and fibrous luminal stenosis, which may represent irreversible panmural fibrosis

From Skinner DB, Belsey RH: Surgical management of esophageal reflux and hiatus hernia: Long-term results with 1,030 patients. J Thorac Cardiovasc Surg 1967; 53:33.

SAVARY AND MILLER CLASSIFICATION

STAGE	DESCRIPTION
I	One or more nonconfluent longitudinal mucosal erosions
II	Confluent ulcerations that do not cover the entire circumference
III	Erosive esophagitis with exudative lesions covering the entire esophageal circumference but without an associated stricture
IV	Chronic changes of reflux including stricture, ulceration, Barrett's mucosa

From Savary M, Miller G: The Esophagus: Handbook and Atlas of Endoscopy. Solothurn, Switzerland: A.G. Gassman, 1978.

Endoscopy of the esophagus for esophagitis is a very common procedure, and these two staging systems make for more accurate descriptions than "mild, moderate, and severe." Which system is used should be clearly identified in the endoscopy report.

GRADING SYSTEM FOR ESOPHAGEAL CAUSTIC INJURIES

GRADE	DESCRIPTION
I	Hyperemia with superficial desquamation
II	Shallow ulcers limited to extent of mucosa, white discoloration of mucosa, often in a linear streaking distribution
III	Deep ulcerations into muscle, may be transluminal

Treatment depends on the grade of injury. Most injuries are Grade I and can be treated without surgery. Treatment of Grade II injuries may involve medications, including steroids, and surgery for complications. Surgery is much more likely for Grade III injuries; when this diagnosis is made at endoscopy, the procedure should be stopped to prevent any further damage.

From Teitelbaum D, Coran A: Caustic burn of the esophagus. In Cameron JL (ed): Current Surgical Therapy, 5th ed. St. Louis: Mosby, 1995:41.

WORLD HEALTH ORGANIZATION CLASSIFICATION OF THYROID GOITER

STAGE	DESCRIPTION
0-A	No goiter
0-B	Goiter detectable by palpation but not visible even with neck fully extended
I	Goiter palpable and visible only with neck fully extended
II	Goiter visible with neck in normal position
III	Large goiter that can be seen at a distance

From Cameron JL (ed): Current Surgical Therapy, 5th ed. St. Louis: Mosby, 1995:511.

CLASSIFICATION OF HYPOTHYROIDISM BY LEVEL OF LESION

	HYPOTHALMUS	PITUITARY	THYROID
Serum TSH	Low	Low	High
Serum TSH after TRH stimulation	Increased	No response	Exaggerated increase
Thyroid response to exogenous TSH	Increased	Increased	No response

TRH, thyroid-releasing hormone; TSH, thyroid-stimulating hormone.

From Sabiston DC (ed): Textbook of Surgery, 14th ed. Philadelphia: W.B. Saunders, 1991:566.

CLASSIFICATION OF NONTOXIC GOITER

TYPE I—NONTOXIC DIFFUSE GOITER
A. Endemic
  1. Iodine deficiency
  2. Iodine excess
  3. Dietary goitrogens
B. Sporadic
  1. Congenital defect in thyroid hormone biosynthesis
  2. Chemical agents (lithium, thiocyanate)
  3. Iodine deficiency
C. Compensatory following subtotal thyroidectomy
TYPE II—NONTOXIC NODULAR GOITER DUE TO CAUSES LISTED
A. Uninodular or multinodular
B. Functional, nonfunctional, or both

From Burrow GN: Nontoxic goiter—diffuse and nodular. In Burrow GN, Oppenheimer JH, Volpe R (eds): Thyroid Function and Disease. Philadelphia: W.B. Saunders, 1989.

CLASSIFICATION OF GASTRIC ULCERS

TYPE	LOCATION
I	Located in the body of the stomach, primarily along the lesser curvature
II	Two ulcers, one prepyloric associated with a second duodenal ulcer
III	Prepyloric location
IV	Near the gastroesophageal junction

Type I and IV ulcers are treated just as gastric ulcers and are thought not to be related to acid hypersecretion, unlike Type II and III ulcers, which must be treated with acid-reducing procedures.

From Cameron JL (ed): Current Surgical Therapy, 5th ed. St. Louis: Mosby, 1995:56.

CLASSIFICATION OF PERIANAL ABSCESS

The classification of a perianal abscess is anatomic. There are five abscesses that classically present:
Superficial perianal
Perirectal
   Ischiorectal (ischioanal)
   Intersphincteric
   Postanal (deep space of Courtney)
   Supralevator

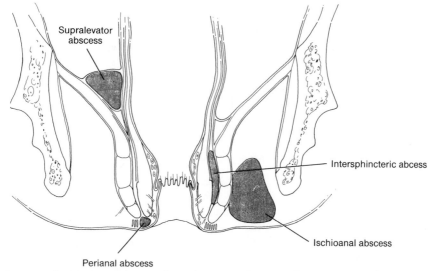

Supralevator abscess

Intersphincteric abcess

Ischioanal abscess

Perianal abscess

Primary distinction to be made is that supralevator abscesses must be drained into the rectum/anus.

Text from Cameron JL (ed): Current Surgical Therapy, 5th ed. St. Louis: Mosby, 1995:225.
Illustration from Gordon PH, Nivatvongs S: Principles and Practice of Surgery for the Colon, Rectum, and Anus. St. Louis: Quality Medical Publishing, 1992:228.

CLASSIFICATION OF INFLAMMATORY BOWEL DISEASE

CHARACTERISTICS	CROHN'S DISEASE	ULCERATIVE COLITIS
A. SIGNS AND SYMPTOMS		
1. Diarrhea	70%–90%	80%–90%
2. Rectal bleeding	Less common	Prominent
3. Abdominal pain	Moderate to severe	Mild
4. Palpable mass	Occasionally	No
5. Anal complaints	Frequent (50%)	Infrequent (<20%)
B. RADIOGRAPHIC FINDINGS		
1. Ileal disease	Common	Rare
2. Nodularity	No	Yes
3. Distribution	Skip areas	Rectum extending upward
4. Ulcer	Linear, cobblestone	Collar button
5. Toxic dilatation	Yes	Yes
C. PROCTOSCOPIC FINDINGS		
1. Anal fissure, fistula, and abscess	Common	Rare
2. Rectal sparing	Common (50%)	Rare
3. Granularity	No	Yes
4. Ulceration	Linear, deep	Superficial erosion

Often inflammatory bowel disease cannot be clearly classified as either ulcerative colitis or Crohn's disease. There is probably a continuum of disease, with some cases representing a combination of the two. Distinction, however, can be important because of differences in management, outcome of surgery, and prognosis.

From Sabiston DC (ed): Textbook of Surgery, 14th ed. Philadelphia: W.B. Saunders, 1991:847.

CLASSIFICATION OF ANORECTAL FISTULAS

TYPE	DESCRIPTION
I	Intersphincteric, the most common, in which the fistulous tract is confined to the intersphincteric plane
II	Trans-sphincteric, in which the fistula connects the intersphincteric plane with the ischiorectal fossa by perforating the external sphincter
III	Suprasphincteric, similar to Type II, but the tract loops over the external sphincter and perforates the levator ani
IV	Extrasphincteric, in which the tract passes from rectum to perineal skin completely external to the sphincteric complex

From Marks CG, Ritchie JK: Anal fistulas at St. Mark's Hospital. Br J Surg 1977; 64:84.

CLASSIFICATION OF RECTOVAGINAL FISTULA

TYPE	LOCATION	ETIOLOGY	SIZE
Simple	Low	Infection, trauma	Small (<2.5 cm)
Complex	High	Inflammatory bowel disease, radiation, cancer	Large (>2.5 cm)

The most common cause of a simple rectovaginal fistula is obstetric injury. Patients complain of the passage of stool or air through the vagina, recurrent vaginitis, and incontinence.

From Cameron JL (ed): Current Surgical Therapy, 4th ed. St. Louis: Mosby, 1992:244.

CLASSIFICATION OF HEMORRHOIDS

DEGREE	DESCRIPTION
1st	Hemorrhoids protrude into the lumen, are visible on anoscopy, but do not prolapse outside the anal canal
2nd	Hemorrhoids prolapse outside the anal canal upon straining but reduce spontaneously
3rd	Hemorrhoids protrude upon straining and must be reduced manually
4th	Hemorrhoids cannot be reduced

Internal hemorrhoids arise above the dentate line and tend to present with bleeding and prolapse, whereas external hemorrhoids are innervated and tend to be painful. Remember that colon cancer should be ruled out first, in most cases, before attributing rectal bleeding solely to hemorrhoids.

From Cameron JL (ed): Current Surgical Therapy, 5th ed. St. Louis: Mosby, 1995:217.

HINCHEY CLASSIFICATION OF PERFORATED DIVERTICULITIS

STAGE	DESCRIPTION
I	The colonic abscess is confined by the mesentery of the colon.
II	There is a pelvic abscess resulting from local perforation of a pericolic abscess.
III	Generalized peritonitis has resulted from a rupture of a pericolonic and pelvic abscess into the peritoneal cavity.
IV	Fecal peritonitis has resulted from free perforation of a diverticulum.

This classification system is useful in determining initial management. Stages I and II can be managed medically initially as long as the patient responds to therapy. Stages III and IV should be explored operatively once adequate resuscitation has been provided.

From Sackier JM: Colonic surgery for acute conditions: Perforated diverticular disease. In Fielding LP, Goldberg SM (eds): Rob and Smith's Operative Surgery: Surgery of the Colon, Rectum and Anus, 5th ed. Oxford: Butterworth-Heinemann, 1993:388.

CLASSIFICATION OF CAUSES OF IMMUNE THROMBOCYTOPENIC PURPURA (ITP)

TYPE I—CONGENITAL

A. Immune
   1. Drug induced
   2. Autoimmune neonatal thrombocytopenia
   3. Maternal antibody-induced neonatal thrombocytopenia
   4. Infection
B. Nonimmune
   1. Drug induced
   2. Erythroblastosis hemangioma
   3. Infection
   4. Giant cavernous hemangioma

TYPE II—ACQUIRED

A. Immune
   1. Drug induced
   2. Sepsis
   3. Post-transfusion purpura
   4. Allergic reaction
   5. Acute or chronic autoimmune thrombocytopenia
B. Nonimmune
   1. Drug induced
   2. Disseminated intravascular coagulation (DIC)
   3. Thrombotic thrombocytopenic purpura (TTP)
   4. Acquired immunodeficiency syndrome (AIDS)

From Koller CA: Immune thrombocytopenic purpura. Med Clin North Am 1980; 64:761–773.

CLASSIFICATION OF STATISTICAL ERRORS

TYPE	DESCRIPTION
I	The null hypothesis has been rejected although it is true
II	The null hypothesis has not been rejected although it is not true

From Blackbourne L, Fleischer K: Advanced Surgical Recall. Baltimore: Williams & Wilkins, 1997:266.

CLASSIFICATION OF POISONOUS SNAKES INDIGENOUS TO THE UNITED STATES

COMMON NAME	IDENTIFICATION	CHARACTERISTICS
Large rattlesnake (diamondback, mojave, timber sidewinder, pacific, prairie)	Broad head, many coloration patterns, light belly; often has diamond markings. Rattles; up to 6 feet in length.	Can strike long distance. Potent cytotoxic venom. Accounts for most severe bites and fatalities.
Small rattlesnake (pigmy, massasauga)	Less than 3 feet in length.	Rattlers often small and audible only at close range. Bites cause severe pain, swelling, few fatalities.
Copperhead	Pink, russet, or orange-brown with dark brown or reddish crossbands. Head is triangular, yellow to copper with pale sides. Two to three feet in length.	Accounts for most bites in eastern United States. Fatalities almost unknown.
Cottonmouth	Olive or brown with wide black crossbands. Yellow belly marked with gray. White interior of mouth. Around 4 feet in length.	Semiaquatic. Belligerent, aggressive behavior. Rare fatalities, but severe tissue destruction by venom.
Coral snake	Complete rings of yellow, black, red, and sometimes white with red and yellow adjacent. Less than 4 feet in length.	Frequently bites are not envenomated. Little local reaction at bite site, but neurotoxin-induced respiratory paralysis in several hours is usually fatal.

The first four snake types belong to the family Crotalidae, *whereas the coral snake is in the family* Elapidae.

From Sabiston DC (ed): Textbook of Surgery, 14th ed. Philadelphia: W.B. Saunders, 1991:250.

CLASSIFICATION OF SNAKE BITE VENENATION

GRADE	DEFINITION	LOCAL SYMPTOMS AND SIGNS	SYSTEMIC SYMPTOMS AND SIGNS
0	No venenation	Fang or tooth marks, minimal pain; edema or erythema of less than 1 inch in 12 hours	None
1	Minimal venenation	Fang or tooth marks, severe pain, 1 to 5 inches of surrounding edema in the first 12 hours	None
2	Moderate venenation	Fang or tooth marks, severe pain, 6 to 12 inches of surrounding edema and erythema in 12 hours	Neurotoxic symptoms, nausea, giddiness, shock, palpable regional lymph nodes
3	Severe venenation	Fang or tooth marks, severe pain, more than 12 inches of surrounding edema and erythema	Hypotension, generalized petechiae and ecchymoses, shock
4	Very severe venenation	Multiple fang or tooth marks; local edema may be present beyond involved extremity to ipsilateral trunk	Always including renal failure, coma, and blood-tinged secretions

From Parrish HM: Incidence of treated snakebites in the United States. Public Health Rep 1966; 81:269.

TANNER STAGES OF FEMALE BREAST DEVELOPMENT

STAGE	BREAST DEVELOPMENT	DESCRIPTION
1		Preadolescent
2		Breast and papilla elevated as small mound; areolar diameter increased
3		Breast and areola enlarged; no contour separation
4		Areola and papilla form secondary mound
5		Mature; nipple projects; areola part of general breast contour

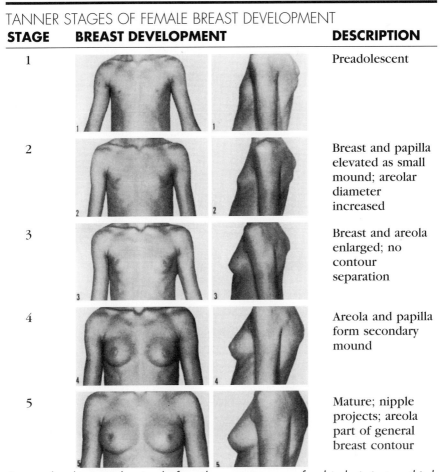

Breast development begins before the appearance of pubic hair in two thirds of girls, and the breasts do not always develop at the same rate.

From Seidel HM, Ball JW, Dains JE, Benedict GW: **Mosby's Guide to Physical Examination.**
St. Louis: Mosby, 1987:79.

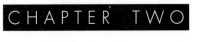
Vascular Surgery

AORTIC DISSECTION CLASSIFICATION

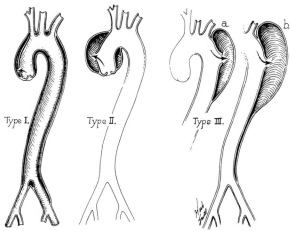

DEBAKEY CLASSIFICATION

TYPE	DESCRIPTION
I	Involvement of the ascending, transverse arch, and descending thoracic aorta, frequently extending into the abdominal aorta
II	Arises in the ascending aorta but terminates just proximal to the origin of the innominate artery
IIIA	Begins just distal to the left subclavian artery and terminates above the diaphragm
IIIB	Begins just distal to the left subclavian artery and extends into the abdominal aorta

STANFORD CLASSIFICATION

TYPE	DESCRIPTION
A	Involves the ascending aorta
B	Does not involve the ascending aorta; arises just distal to the left subclavian

*Aortic dissection involving the ascending aorta is a surgical emergency.
Aortic dissection involving the descending aorta, if it takes off below the left subclavian, usually can be managed medically.*

From DeBakey ME, Lawrie GM, Crawford ES, et al.: Surgical treatment of dissecting aortic aneurysms: 28 years experience with 527 cases. Contemporary Surgery 1984; 25:13.

CLASSIFICATION OF TAKAYASU'S ARTERITIS

TYPE	DESCRIPTION
I	Involvement of the arch and the take-off of the three main branches
II	Involvement of the descending aorta, including the intraabdominal portion
III	Involvement of the aortic arch and descending aorta, including the intraabdominal portion
IV	Involvement of the pulmonary vasculature

From Ueno A, Awane Y, Wakabayashi A, Shimizu K: Successfully operated obliterative brachiocephalic arteritis (Takayasu) associated with the elongated coarctation. Jpn Heart J 1967; 8:538.

CLASSIFICATION OF EXTREMITY OUTFLOW OBSTRUCTION

GRADE	CLINICAL STATE	PRESSURE CHANGE AT REST	HYPEREMIA PRESSURE CHANGE
I	Fully compensated	<4	<6
II	Partially compensated	<4	>6
III	Partially decompensated	>4	>6
IV	Fully decompensated	15–20	No further increase

From Raju S: New approaches to the diagnosis and treatment of venous obstruction. J Vasc Surg 1986; 4:42.

STAGES OF ARTERIAL THORACIC OUTLET SYNDROME

STAGE	DESCRIPTION
0	Asymptomatic cervical rib with no subclavian artery enlargement: no treatment required
I	Asymptomatic cervical rib with poststenotic dilatation less than twice the subclavian arterial diameter: cervial rib is resected, but the artery is left alone
II	Cervical rib with aneurysm, intimal damage, and mural thrombosis: rib is resected and artery repaired by excision and end-to-end anastomosis or bypass graft
III	Cervical rib with distal emboli: rib is resected, artery repaired or replaced, and embolectomy performed down to the elbow; intraoperative thrombolysis may be tried for emboli in the hand or forearm; dorsal sympathectomy is added for ischemia and gangrene

From Cameron JL (ed): Current Surgical Therapy, 5th ed. St. Louis: Mosby, 1995:737.

CLINICAL CLASSIFICATION OF CEREBROVASCULAR DISEASE (CHAT)

CLASS	CURRENT CLINICAL STATE (C)	PAST HISTORY (H)	ARTERY (A)	TARGET ORGAN (T)
0	Asymptomatic	Asymptomatic	No lesion	No lesion
1	TIA	TIA	Appropriate lesion	Appropriate lesion
2	Temporary stroke	Temporary stroke	Lesion in other vascular territory	Lesion in other vascular territory
3	Permanent stroke	Permanent stroke	Appropriate lesion and lesion in other territory	Appropriate lesion and lesion in other territory
4	Nonspecific dysfunction	Nonspecific dysfunction		
5	Changing stroke			

TIA, transient ischemic attack.

From Rutherford RB: Vascular Surgery, 3rd ed. Philadelphia: W.B. Saunders, 1989:398.

CLASSIFICATION OF PORTAL HYPERTENSION BY SITE OF OBSTRUCTION

TYPE 1—PRESINUSOIDAL OBSTRUCTION
A. Extrahepatic
   1. Portal vein thrombosis
   2. Congenital atresia
   3. Neonatal omphalitis
   4. Pylephlebitis
   5. Hypercoagulable states
   6. Stasis
   7. Trauma
   8. Adjacent inflammation
   9. Mechanical obstruction
B. Intrahepatic
   1. Schistosomiasis
   2. Congenital hepatic fibrosis
   3. Hepatoportal sclerosis
   4. Myeloproliferative disorders
   5. Sarcoidosis
   6. Gaucher's disease
   7. Arsenic toxicity
   8. Primary biliary cirrhosis

TYPE II—SINUSOIDAL OBSTRUCTION
A. Fatty metamorphosis
B. Toxic hepatitis
C. Wilson's disease
D. Cirrhosis

TYPE III—POSTSINUSOIDAL OBSTRUCTION
A. Intrahepatic
   1. Cirrhosis—nutritional, postnecrotic, secondary biliary
   2. Hemochromatosis
   3. Viral hepatitis
   4. Alcoholic hepatitis
   5. Budd-Chiari syndrome
B. Extrahepatic
   1. Budd-Chiari syndrome
   2. Congenital suprahepatic inferior vena cava webs
   3. Hepatic, renal, and adrenal neoplasms
   4. Trauma
   5. Sepsis
   6. Cardiac causes—constrictive pericarditis, congestive heart failure

TYPE IV—HIGH FLOW PORTAL HYPERTENSION
A. Arteriovenous
B. Hepatic artery/portal vein
C. Splenic
D. Mesenteric
E. Massive splenomegaly

From Rutherford RB: Vascular Surgery, 3rd ed. Philadelphia: W.B. Saunders, 1989:1117.

CLASSIFICATION OF VENOUS VALVULAR INCOMPETENCE BY DESCENDING PHLEBOGRAPHY

GRADE	VALVE CONDITION	REFLUX LEVEL OF CONTRAST MATERIAL	
		Normal Breathing	Valsalva
0	Competent	None	None
I	Minimal	Upper thigh	NA
II	Mild	Knee	Increased
III	Moderate	Below knee	Increased
IV	Severe	Ankle	NA

NA, not applicable.

From Rutherford RB: Vascular Surgery, 3rd ed. Philadelphia: W.B. Saunders, 1989:1616.

CRAWFORD CLASSIFICATION OF THORACOABDOMINAL AORTIC ANEURYSMS

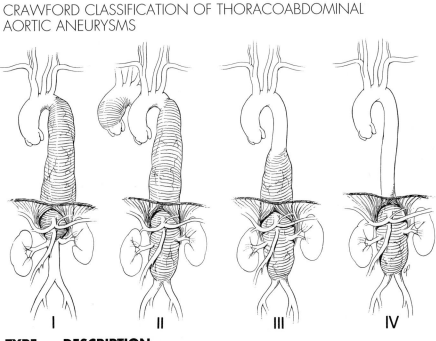

I   II   III   IV

TYPE	DESCRIPTION
I	Involves all of the descending thoracic aorta and extends down to the visceral vessels in the abdomen
II	Extends from the left subclavian artery to the aortic bifurcation
III	Involves the distal half of the descending thoracic aorta and most or all of the abdominal aorta
IV	Begins near the diaphragm and usually extends to the aortic bifurcation

From Cameron JL (ed): Current Surgical Therapy, 5th ed. St. Louis: Mosby, 1995:625–626.

GRADING SYSTEM OF PERIPHERAL ISCHEMIA

GRADE	DESCRIPTION
I	Viable extremity, no muscle weakness, no sensory loss, audible arterial and venous pulses by Doppler, and intact capillary refill
II	Salvageable extremity, mild muscle weakness and sensory loss, inaudible arterial pulse but audible venous pulse by Doppler, slow capillary refill
III	Irreversible damage to extremity with muscle paralysis, anesthetic extremity, inaudible arterial and venous pulses by Doppler, and absent capillary refill

Patients with acute ischemia present with the well-known five Ps—pain, paresthesias, pulselessness, pallor, and paralysis. Those patients presenting with Grade III ischemia need immediate restoration of blood flow without any delay.

From Suggested standards for reports dealing with lower extremity ischemia. J Vasc Surg 1986; 4:80–94.

CLINICAL CLASSIFICATION OF CHRONIC VENOUS INSUFFICIENCY (CVI)

STAGE	SYMPTOMS AND SIGNS
0	Asymptomatic
I	Mild CVI with complaints of limb swelling or aching
II	Moderate CVI with significant hyperpigmentation and other skin changes but no ulceration
III	Severe CVI with skin changes and an active or recently healed ulcer

From Cameron JL (ed): Current Surgical Therapy, 5th ed. St. Louis: Mosby, 1995:749.

CLASSIFICATION OF AORTOILIAC OCCLUSIVE DISEASE

TYPE	DESCRIPTION
I	Localized disease confined to the distal aorta and common iliac arteries
II	More widespread intraabdominal disease
III	Signifies multilevel disease with associated infrainguinal occlusive lesions

From Dean RH, Yao JST, Brewster DC (eds): Current Diagnosis and Treatment in Vascular Surgery. Norwalk, CT: Appleton & Lange, 1995:197.

CLASSIFICATION OF PULMONARY THROMBOEMBOLISM

CLASS	SYMPTOMS	ARTERIAL GASES	% PA OCCLUSION	HEMODYNAMICS
I	None	Normal	<20	Normal
II	Anxiety Hyperventilation	$Pao_2<80$ mm Hg $Paco_2<35$ mm Hg	20–30	Tachycardia
III	Dyspnea Collapse	$Pao_2<65$ mm Hg $Paco_2<30$ mm Hg	30–50	CVP elevated PAP>20 mm Hg
IV	Shock Dyspnea	$Pao_2<50$ mm Hg $Paco_2<30$ mm Hg	>50	CVP elevated PAP>25 mm Hg SBP<100 mm Hg
V	Dyspnea Syncope	$Pao_2<50$ mm Hg $Paco_2>30$ mm Hg	>50	CVP elevated PAP>40 mm Hg CO low No shock

CO, cardiac output; CVP, central venous pressure; PA, pulmonary artery; PAP, mean pulmonary artery pressure; SBP, systolic blood pressure. *From Greenfield L: Venous and lymphatic disease. In Schwartz SI (ed): Principles of Surgery. New York: McGraw-Hill, 1989:1024.*

CLASSIFICATION OF LOWER EXTREMITY BLOOD FLOW BY ANKLE-BRACHIAL INDEX (ABI)

ABI	CLINICAL CORRELATION
>1.0	Diabetic extremity with calcified blood vessels yielding a falsely high index of perfusion
1.0–0.7	No symptoms of vascular disease
0.7–0.5	Claudication (pain in the extremity following ambulation)
<0.3	Rest pain, ulcer, or gangrene

The ankle-brachial index (ABI) is the ratio of systolic blood pressure in the lower extremity to the systolic blood pressure in the upper extremity.

From Dean RH, Yao JST, Brewster DC (eds): **Current Diagnosis and Treatment in Vascular Surgery. Norwalk, CT: Appleton & Lange, 1995:2–3.**

GRADING OF ARTERIAL PULSATIONS

GRADE	DESCRIPTION
4+	Pulse is normal
3+	Pulse is slightly diminished
2+	Pulse is markedly diminished
1+	Pulse is barely palpable
0	Pulse is absent

Some vascular surgeons find it difficult to reproducibly distinguish between "slightly" and "markedly" diminished pulses, and therefore employ a 2-1-0 system in which the pulse is either present, diminished, or absent. If there is confusion, it may be helpful to describe the pulse as 2/4 or 2/2, and thus clarify which grading system is being used.

From Way LW (ed): **Current Surgical Diagnosis and Treatment, 9th ed. Norwalk, CT: Appleton & Lange, 1991:728.**

CHAPTER THREE

Cardiothoracic Surgery

CLASSIFICATION OF TRUNCUS ARTERIOSUS

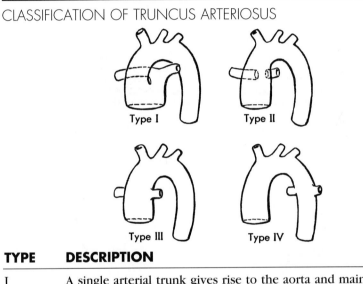

Type I	Type II

Type III	Type IV

TYPE	DESCRIPTION
I	A single arterial trunk gives rise to the aorta and main pulmonary artery
II	The right and left pulmonary arteries arise immediately adjacent to one another from the dorsal wall of the truncus
III	The right and left pulmonary arteries arise from either side of the truncus
IV	The proximal pulmonary arteries are absent and pulmonary blood flow is by way of bronchial arteries

From Keith JD, Rowe RD, Vlad P: Heart Disease in Infancy and Childhood. New York: Macmillan, 1958:521.

CLASSIFICATION OF PULMONARY ARTERIOVENOUS MALFORMATIONS

TYPE	DESCRIPTION
I	Multiple small arteriovenous fistulae without aneurysm
II	Large single arteriovenous aneurysm—peripheral
IIIa	Large single arteriovenous aneurysm—central
IIIb	Large arteriovenous aneurysm with anomalous venous drainage
IIIc	Multiple small arteriovenous fistulae with anomalous venous drainage
IVa	Large single venous aneurysm with systemic artery communication
IVb	Large single venous aneurysm without fistula—varix of pulmonary vein
V	Anomalous venous drainage without fistula

From Anabtawi IN, Ellison RG, Ellison LT: Pulmonary arteriovenous aneurysms and fistulas: Anatomic variations, embryology, and classification. Ann Thorac Surg 1965; 1:277.

ANGIOGRAPHIC GRADING OF CARDIAC VALVULAR REGURGITATION

I. Aortic Regurgitation

GRADE	DESCRIPTION
1+	Small jet of contrast into LV that clears with each beat
2+	Moderate opacification of LV, but less than aorta; incomplete clearing with each beat
3+	Persistent marked opacification of LV, equal to aorta after three beats
4+	Persistent marked opacification of LV, equal to aorta within three beats

II. Mitral Regurgitation

GRADE	DESCRIPTION
1+	Small jet of contrast into LA that clears with each beat
2+	Moderate opacification of LA, but less than LV; incomplete clearing of each beat
3+	Persistent marked opacification of LA, equal to LV after three beats
4+	Persistent marked opacification of LA, equal to LV within three beats; systolic reflux into pulmonary veins may be observed

LA, left atrium; LV, left ventricle.

From Sabiston DC (ed): Textbook of Surgery, 14th ed. Philadelphia: W.B. Saunders, 1991:1836.

CLASSIFICATION OF THE HYPOPLASTIC LEFT HEART SYNDROME

CLASS	DESCRIPTION
I	Isolated cardiac anomaly
II	Two congenital anomalies affecting left ventricular outflow
III	More than two anomalies, or two with coexisting left ventricular or ascending aortic or aortic arch hypoplasia
IV	Aortic atresia

The syndrome consists of congenital mitral valve disease; left ventricular hypoplasia (with concordant ventriculoarterial connection); subvalvar, valvar, or supravalvar aortic stenosis; ascending aortic or arch hypoplasia; interrupted aortic arch; or coarctation.

From Kirklin JW, Barratt-Boyes BG: Cardiac Surgery, 2nd ed. New York: Churchill Livingstone, 1993:1269.

CLASSIFICATION OF BRONCHIECTASIS

TYPE	DESCRIPTION
Postinfection saccular bronchiectasis	Related to pertussis, bacterial and viral pneumonia, bronchial stricture, foreign body
Cylindric bronchiectasis	Related to pulmonary infection, chronic aspiration
Pseudobronchiectasis	No true bronchiectasis
Post-tuberculous bronchiectasis	Bronchiectasis following tuberculosis infection
Genetic related bronchiectasis	

From Hood RM: Bacterial infections of the lungs. In Shields TW (ed): General Thoracic Surgery, 4th ed. Philadelphia: Lippincott-Raven, 1994:930.

STAGING OF PULMONARY NON-HODGKIN'S LYMPHOMA

STAGE	EXTENT OF DISEASE
I_E	Lung only involved
II_E	Lung and hilar nodes involved
II_{2E}	Lung and mediastinal nodes involved
II_{2EW}	Lung and adjacent chest wall or diaphragm involved
III and IV	Disseminated disease

From L'hoste RJ, et al.: Primary pulmonary lymphoma. Cancer 1984; 54:1397.

STAGING OF KAWASAKI'S DISEASE

STAGE	DURATION	SYMPTOMS	PATHOLOGY
I	0-9 days	Fever Conjunctivitis Mucocutaneous changes	Myocarditis Perivasculitis of arterioles, capillaries, and venules Intimal inflammation of medium and large arterioles
II	10-20 days	Fever Palpable aneurysms	Panvasculitis Coronary and peripheral aneurysms, with early thrombosis
III	21-31 days	Arthritis	Coronary aneurysms Thrombosis and stenosis
IV	>40 days	Angina	Scarring, fibrosis, and intimal thickening

Kawasaki's disease is a pansystemic disorder of undetermined cause that primarily affects infants and children, leading in rare cases to severe cardiac disease. Management consists of antiplatelet drugs and intravenous immunoglobulin.

From Fujiwara H, Hamashima Y: Pathology of the heart in Kawasaki disease. Pediatrics 1978; 61:100.

STAGING OF THYMOMAS

STAGE	DESCRIPTION
I	Completely encapsulated, no capsular invasion
II	Invasion into surrounding fatty tissue, mediastinal pleura, or capsule
III	Invasion into neighboring structure (pericardium, lung, great vessels)
IVA	Pleural, pericardial metastasis
IVB	Lymphogenous or hematogenous metastasis

From Trastek VF, Payne WS: Surgery of the thymus gland. In Shields TW (ed): General Thoracic Surgery, 3rd ed. Philadelphia: Lea & Febiger, 1989.

CLASSIFICATION OF BENIGN ESOPHAGEAL TUMORS

TYPE I—INTRALUMINAL
a. Polyps
   1a. Fibrolipoma
   2a. Fibrovascular
   3a. Fibroneuroid
TYPE II—SUBMUCOSAL
a. Hemangioma
b. Granular cell myoblastoma
TYPE III—INTRAMURAL
a. Leiomyoma
b. Duplication
c. Cyst

From Murray GF, Gustafson RA: Benign tumors, cysts, and duplications of the esophagus. In Shields TW (ed): General Thoracic Surgery, 4th ed. Philadelphia: Lippincott-Raven, 1994:1622.

ENDOSCOPIC GRADING OF CORROSIVE BURNS OF THE ESOPHAGUS AND STOMACH

GRADE	PATHOLOGY	ENDOSCOPIC FINDINGS
First degree	Superficial involvement of mucosa	Mucosal hyperemia and edema
Second degree	Transmucosal involvement with or without involvement of muscularis	Sloughing of mucosa
	No extension into the periesophageal or perigastric tissue	Hemorrhages, exudates, and ulceration, pseudomembrane formation, and granulation tissue if examined late
Third degree	Full thickness injuries with extension into the periesophageal or perigastric tissues	Sloughing of tissues with deep ulcerations
	Mediastinal or intraperitoneal organs may be involved	Complete obliteration of esophageal lumen by massive edema; charring and eschar formation, full thickness necrosis with perforation

From Estrera A, et al.: Corrosive burns of the esophagus and stomach: A recommendation for an aggressive surgical approach. Ann Thorac Surg 1986; 41:276.

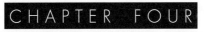

CHAPTER FOUR

Trauma and Burn Surgery

HEMORRHAGIC SHOCK CLASSIFICATION

SIGN	CLASS			
	I	**II**	**III**	**IV**
Blood loss	<15% blood volume	15%–30%	30%–40%	>40%
Heart rate	<100	>100	>120	>140
Blood pressure	Normal	Normal	Decreased	Decreased
Pulse pressure	Normal or widened	Narrowed	Narrowed	Very narrow
Capillary refill	Normal	Delayed	Delayed	Delayed
Skin	Normal	Cool, pale	Cool, pale	Cold, ashen, mottled
Respiratory rate	14–20	20–30	30–40	>35
Urine output	>30 mL/hr	20–30	5–15	Negligible
Mental status	Slightly anxious	Mildly anxious, thirsty	Anxious, confused	Lethargy, coma

One of the first signs of hypovolemia in the trauma patient is tachycardia.

*From **Advanced Trauma Life Support Program for Physicians.** Instructor manual. Chicago: American College of Surgeons, 1993:86.*

VAGINA INJURY SCALE

GRADE	DESCRIPTION
I	Contusion/hematoma
II	Superficial laceration (skin only)
III	Deep laceration (into adjacent fat/muscle)
IV	Laceration—complex into cervix
V	Injury into adjacent organs (anus, rectum, urethra, bladder)

*From **Organ Injury Scaling Committee, American Association for the Surgery of Trauma.***

ADVANCED TRAUMA LIFE SUPPORT (ATLS) COURSE WOUND CLASSIFICATION

CLINICAL FEATURES	NONTETANUS-PRONE	TETANUS-PRONE
Age of wound	<6 hrs	>6 hrs
Configuration	Linear	Stellate, avulsion, abrasion
Depth	<1 cm	>1 cm
Mechanism	Sharp surface (knife)	Missile, crush, burn, frostbite
Signs of infection	Absent	Present
Devitalized tissue	Absent	Present
Contaminants (Dirt, feces)	Absent	Present
Ischemic tissue	Absent	Present

When in doubt, give tetanus prophylaxis to trauma patients.

From **Advanced Trauma Life Support Program For Physicians.** *Instructor manual. Chicago:* *American College of Surgeons, 1993:366.*

UTERUS (NONPREGNANT) INJURY SCALE

GRADE	DESCRIPTION
I	Contusion/hematoma
II	Superficial laceration (<1 cm)
III	Deep laceration (>1 cm)
IV	Laceration involving uterine artery
V	Avulsion/devascularization

UTERUS (PREGNANT) INJURY SCALE

GRADE	DESCRIPTION
I	Contusion/hematoma (without placental abruption)
II	Superficial laceration (<1 cm) or partial placental abruption (<25%)
III	Deep laceration (>1 cm) or placental abruption (25%–50%)
IV	Laceration involving uterine artery; deep laceration (>1 cm) with 50% placental abruption
V	Uterine rupture; complete placental abruption

From **Organ Injury Scaling Committee, American Association for the Surgery of Trauma.**

LIVER INJURY SCALE

GRADE	DESCRIPTION
I	Hematoma: subcapsular, nonexpanding, <10% surface area Laceration: capsular tear, nonbleeding, <1 cm parenchymal depth
II	Hematoma: subcapsular, nonexpanding, 10%–50% surface area; intraparenchymal, nonexpanding, <10 cm diameter Laceration: capsular tear, active bleeding, 1–3 cm parenchymal depth, <10 cm in length
III	Hematoma: subcapsular, >50% surface area or expanding ruptured subcapsular hematoma with active bleeding; intraparenchymal hematoma >10 cm or expanding Laceration: >3 cm parenchymal depth
IV	Hematoma: ruptured intraparenchymal hematoma with active bleeding Laceration: parenchymal disruption involving 25%–75% of hepatic lobe or 1–3 Couinaud's segments within a single lobe
V	Laceration: parenchymal disruption involving >75% of hepatic lobe or >3 Couinaud's segments within a lobe Vascular: juxtahepatic venous injuries (retrohepatic vena cava/major hepatic veins)
VI	Vascular: hepatic avulsion

Advance one grade for multiple injuries up to Grade III.
Grade I and II injuries may be managed nonoperatively in the stable patient.
Remember that nonoperative management is not "conservative" and requires close monitoring of the patient.

From Organ Injury Scaling Committee, American Association for the Surgery of Trauma.

BLADDER INJURY SCALE

GRADE	DESCRIPTION
I	Hematoma: contusion, intramural hematoma Laceration: partial thickness
II	Laceration: extraperitoneal bladder wall laceration <2 cm
III	Laceration: extraperitoneal (>2 cm) or intraperitoneal (<2 cm) bladder wall lacerations
IV	Laceration: intraperitoneal bladder wall laceration >2 cm
V	Laceration: intra- or extraperitoneal bladder wall laceration extending into the bladder neck or ureteral orifice (trigone)

Advance one grade for multiple injuries to the same organ.

From Organ Injury Scaling Committee, American Association for the Surgery of Trauma.

OVARY INJURY SCALE

GRADE	DESCRIPTION
I	Contusion/hematoma
II	Superficial laceration (<0.5 cm)
III	Deep laceration (>0.5 cm)
IV	Partial disruption of blood supply
V	Avulsion or complete parenchymal destruction

From Organ Injury Scaling Committee, American Association for the Surgery of Trauma.

CLASSIFICATION OF RENAL INJURIES

GRADE	DESCRIPTION
I	Contusion: microscopic or gross hematuria; urologic studies normal
	Hematoma: subcapsular, nonexpanding without parenchymal laceration
II	Hematoma: nonexpanding perirenal hematoma confined to the renal retroperitoneum
	Laceration: <1 cm parenchymal depth of renal cortex without urinary extravasation
III	Laceration: >1 cm parenchymal depth of renal cortex without collecting system rupture or urinary extravasation
IV	Laceration: parenchymal laceration extending through the renal cortex, medulla, and collecting system
	Vascular: main renal artery or vein injury with contained hemorrhage
V	Laceration: completely shattered kidney
	Vascular: avulsion of renal hilum that devascularizes kidney

Advance one grade for multiple injuries to the same organ.

From Organ Injury Scaling Committee, American Association for the Surgery of Trauma.

RECTAL ORGAN INJURY SCALE

GRADE	DESCRIPTION
I	Hematoma: contusion or hematoma without devascularization
	Laceration: partial thickness laceration
II	Laceration: <50% circumferential laceration
III	Laceration: >50% circumferential laceration
IV	Laceration: full-thickness laceration with extension into the perineum
V	Vascular: devascularized segment

Advance one grade for multiple injuries to the same organ.

From Organ Injury Scaling Committee, American Association for the Surgery of Trauma.

COLON INJURY SCALE

GRADE	DESCRIPTION
I	Hematoma: contusion or hematoma without devascularization
	Laceration: partial thickness, no perforation
II	Laceration: <50% circumferential laceration
III	Laceration: >50% circumferential laceration
IV	Laceration: transection of the colon
V	Laceration: transection of the colon with segmental tissue loss

Advance one grade for multiple injuries, up to Grade III.

From Organ Injury Scaling Committee, American Association for the Surgery of Trauma.

PANCREATIC INJURY SCALE

GRADE	DESCRIPTION
I	Hematoma: minor contusion without duct injury
	Laceration: superficial laceration without duct injury
II	Hematoma: major contusion without duct injury or tissue loss
	Laceration: major laceration without duct injury or tissue loss
III	Laceration: distal transection or parenchymal injury with duct injury
IV	Laceration: proximal transection or parenchymal injury not involving ampulla
V	Laceration: massive disruption of pancreatic head

Advance one grade for multiple injuries to the same organ.

From Organ Injury Scaling Committee, American Association for the Surgery of Trauma.

DUODENAL ORGAN INJURY SCALE

GRADE	DESCRIPTION
I	Hematoma: involves single portion of duodenum
	Laceration: partial thickness, no perforation
II	Hematoma: involves more than one portion
	Laceration: disruption <50% of circumference
III	Laceration: disruption of 50%–75% circumference of D2; disruption 50%–100% circumference of D1, D3, or D4
IV	Laceration: disruption >75% circumference of D2; involves ampulla or distal common bile duct
V	Laceration: massive disruption of duodenopancreatic complex
	Vascular: devascularization of duodenum

From Organ Injury Scaling Committee, American Association for the Surgery of Trauma.

SPLENIC INJURY SCALE

GRADE	DESCRIPTION
I	Hematoma: subcapsular, nonexpanding <10% surface area Laceration: capsular tear, nonbleeding, <1 cm parenchymal depth
II	Hematoma: subcapsular, nonexpanding, 10%–50% surface area; intraparenchymal, nonexpanding, <5 cm in diameter Laceration: capsular tear, active bleeding; 1–3 cm parenchymal depth that does not involve a trabecular vessel
III	Hematoma: subcapsular, >50% surface area or expanding; ruptured subcapsular hematoma with active bleeding; intraparenchymal hematoma >5 cm or expanding Laceration: >3 cm parenchymal depth or involving trabecular vessels
IV	Hematoma: ruptured intraparenchymal hematoma with active bleeding Laceration: laceration involving segmental or hilar vessels producing major devascularization (>25% of spleen)
V	Laceration: completely shattered spleen Vascular: splenic devascularization

Advance one grade for multiple injuries, up to Grade III.
Grade I injuries require little or no treatment. Higher grade injuries in the stable patient may be treated with close observation, especially in the pediatric population.

From Organ Injury Scaling Committee, American Association for the Surgery of Trauma.

EXTRAHEPATIC BILIARY TREE INJURY SCALE

GRADE	DESCRIPTION
I	Gallbladder contusion Portal triad contusion
II	Partial gallbladder avulsion from liver bed; cystic duct intact Laceration or perforation of the gallbladder
III	Complete gallbladder avulsion from liver bed Cystic duct laceration/transection
IV	Partial or complete right hepatic duct laceration Partial or complete left hepatic duct laceration Partial common hepatic duct laceration (<50%) Partial common hepatic bile duct laceration (50%)
V	>50% transection of common hepatic duct >50% transection of common bile duct Intraduodenal, intrapancreatic common bile duct injuries

Advance one grade for multiple injuries, up to Grade III.

From Organ Injury Scaling Committee, American Association for the Surgery of Trauma.

DIAPHRAGM INJURY SCALE

GRADE	DESCRIPTION
I	Contusion
II	Laceration <2 cm
III	Laceration 2-10 cm
IV	Laceration >10 cm with tissue loss <25 cm^2
V	Laceration with tissue loss >25 cm^2

Advance one grade for bilateral injuries, up to Grade III.

From Organ Injury Scaling Committee, American Association for the Surgery of Trauma.

MODIFIED CRAMS SCALE

Circulation	2—Normal capillary refill and BP >100
	1—Delayed capillary refill or BP 85-99
	0—No capillary refill or BP <85
Respiration	2—Normal
	1—Abnormal (labored, shallow, or rate >35)
	0—Absent
Abdomen	2—Abdomen and thorax not tender
	1—Abdomen or thorax tender
	0—Abdomen rigid, thorax flail, or deep penetrating injury to either chest or abdomen
Motor	2—Normal (obeys commands)
	1—Responds only to pain, no posturing
	0—Postures or no response
Speech	2—Normal (oriented)
	1—Confused or inappropriate
	0—Unintelligible or no sounds
	TOTAL = 10-0

BP, blood pressure.

From Clemmer TP, Orme JF, Thomas F, Brooks KA: Prospective evaluation of the CRAMS scale for triaging major trauma. J Trauma 1985; 25:188–191.

NERVE INJURY CLASSIFICATION

DEGREE	ANATOMIC DISRUPTION
1st	Conduction loss only, without anatomic disruption
2nd	Axonal disruption without loss of the neurolemmal sheath
3rd	Loss of axons and nerve sheaths
4th	Fascicular disruption
5th	Nerve transection

From Sunderland S: Nerves and Nerve Injuries. Edinburgh: Churchill Livingstone, 1978:127.

MANGLED EXTREMITY SEVERITY SCORE (MESS)

TYPE	CHARACTERISTICS	INJURIES	POINTS
SKELETAL/ SOFT TISSUE			
1	Low energy	Stab wounds, simple closed fractures, small-caliber gunshot wounds	1
2	Medium energy	Open or multiple-level fractures, 2 dislocations, moderate crush injuries	2
3	High energy	Close-range shotgun blast, high-velocity gunshot wounds	3
4	Massive crush	Logging, oil rig accidents	4
SHOCK			
1	Normotensive hemodynamics	BP stable in field and in OR	0
2	Transiently hypotensive	BP unstable in field but responsive to IV fluids	1
3	Prolonged hypotension	BP <90 in field and responsive to IV fluids only in OR	2
ISCHEMIA			
1	None	Pulsatile limb with ischemia	0[a]
2	Mild	Diminished pulses without signs of ischemia	1[a]
3	Moderate	No pulse by Doppler, sluggish capillary refill, paresthesia, diminished motor activity	2[a]
4	Advanced	Pulseless, cool, paralyzed, and numb without capillary refill	3[a]
AGE			
1	<30 years		0
2	30–50 years		1
3	>50 years		2

TOTAL = 1–11

A total MESS of 7 or more suggests that limb salvage is not possible, although some have questioned this particular grading system.

[a] Points × 2 if ischemia exceeds 6 hours.
BP, blood pressure; IV, intravenous; OR, operating room.

From Johansen K, Daines M, Howey T, et al.: Objective criteria accurately predict amputation following lower extremity trauma. J Trauma 1990; 30:568.

ABBREVIATED INJURY SCALE and INJURY SEVERITY SCORE

The Abbreviated Injury Scale (AIS) was developed in 1969 and is a list of several hundred injuries. Each injury is assigned a number from 1 (minor) to 6 (nearly always fatal). The AIS has been revised multiple times, and recent versions incorporate ICD-9-CM codes.

The Injury Severity Score (ISS) is used to characterize the multiply injured trauma patient. The ISS varies from 1 to 75. A patient with an AIS score of 6 is designated a 75 automatically. If a patient does not have an AIS of 6, the ISS is calculated by adding the squares of the three highest AIS scores for injuries to different body regions. The ISS correlates with mortality.

Example: *A patient with a ruptured spleen, fractured ribs, pulmonary contusion, and femur fracture would have the following ISS:*

Abdomen	Ruptured spleen	AIS 2
Chest	Fractured ribs	AIS 2
	Pulmonary contusion	AIS 3
Extremities	Fractured femur	AIS 3

$$ISS = 2^2 + 3^2 + 3^2 = 22$$

From Feliciano D, et al.: Trauma, 3rd ed. New York: McGraw-Hill, 1996.

REVISED TRAUMA SCORE (Add best in each category together)

Respiratory rate	10–29 = 4
	>29 = 3
	6–9 = 2
	1–5 = 1
	0 = 0
Systolic blood pressure	>89 = 4
	76–89 = 3
	50–75 = 2
	1–49 = 1
	0 = 0
Glasgow Coma Scale	13–15 = 4
	9–12 = 3
	6–8 = 2
	4–5 = 1
	<4 = 0
TOTAL	0–12

The Revised Trauma Score incorporates the Glasgow Coma Scale with two other easily measured parameters. Patients with a high Revised Trauma Score have a greater chance of survival than those with low scores.

From Champion HR, Sacco WJ, Copes WS, et al.: A revision of the Trauma Score. J Trauma 1989; 29:623.

PEDIATRIC TRAUMA SCORE (PTS)

	+2	**+1**	**−1**
Size	>20 kg	10–20 kg	<10 kg
Airway	Normal	Maintained	Unmaintained
Systolic blood pressure	>90	50–90	<50
Central nervous system	Awake	Obtunded	Coma
Open wound	None	Minor	Major
Skeletal	None	Closed	Open—multiple

The PTS ranges from −6 to 12, and children scoring 8 or less should be considered for transport to a pediatric trauma center.

From Feliciano D, et al.: Trauma, 3rd ed. New York: McGraw-Hill, 1996.

LUNG INJURY SCORE

CHEST RADIOGRAPH SCORE	POINTS
No alveolar consolidation	0
Alveolar consolidation confined to one quadrant	1
Alveolar consolidation confined to two quadrants	2
Alveolar consolidation confined to three quadrants	3
Alveolar consolidation confined to four quadrants	4

HYPOXEMIA SCORE

Pao_2/FIo_2 >300	0
Pao_2/FIo_2 225–299	1
Pao_2/FIo_2 175–224	2
Pao_2/FIo_2 100–174	3
Pao_2/FIo_2 <100	4

PEEP SCORE (WHEN VENTILATED)

PEEP < 5 cm H_2O	0
PEEP 6–8 cm H_2O	1
PEEP 9–11 cm H_2O	2
PEEP 12–14 cm H_2O	3
PEEP >14 cm H_2O	4

RESPIRATORY SYSTEM COMPLIANCE SCORE (WHEN AVAILABLE)

Compliance >80 mL/cm H_2O	0
Compliance 60–79 mL/cm H_2O	1
Compliance 40–59 mL/cm H_2O	2
Compliance 20–39 mL/cm H_2O	3
Compliance <20 mL/cm H_2O	4

TOTAL = sum/no. of components used
No lung injury: 0
Mild to moderate lung injury: 0.1–2.5
Severe lung injury (ARDS): >2.5

ARDS, acute respiratory distress syndrome; PEEP, positive end-expiratory pressure.

From Murray JF: Lung injury score. Am Rev Respir Dis 1988; 134:720. © American Lung Association.

GLASGOW COMA SCALE (Add best in each category together)

Eyes	Open spontaneously	4
	Open to verbal command	3
	Open to pain	2
	Do not open	1
Verbal	Oriented, conversing	5
	Disoriented, conversing	4
	Inappropriate words	3
	Incomprehensible sounds	2
	No response	1
Motor	Obeys verbal commands	6
	Localizes pain	5
	Withdraws from pain	4
	Abnormal flexion	3
	Abnormal extension	2
	No response	1
	TOTAL	3-15

The score can be designated as a single number (i.e., GCS 9), or presented as a series of three numbers (i.e., E3V4M5). Patients with a GCS of 8 or less are in a coma and usually require airway placement.

From Lopez-Viego M (ed): The Parkland Trauma Handbook. *St. Louis: Mosby, 1994:30.*

LE FORT'S CLASSIFICATION OF MIDFACE FRACTURES

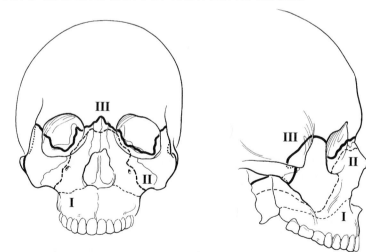

Most fractures of the midface represent combinations of the three classic Le Fort patterns. Any patient with swelling and bruising of the central third of the face should be evaluated for possible midfacial fractures. Treatment involves reduction and stabilization of the individual fractured segments.

From Marks MW, Marks C (eds): Fundamentals of Plastic Surgery. *Philadelphia: W.B. Saunders, 1997:214.*

CRITICAL CARE UNIT CLASSIFICATION

CLASS	PHYSICIAN COVERAGE	NURSE:PATIENT RATIO	MONITORING
I	Present in ICU	1 : 1 or 1 : 2	Invasive
II	Present in hospital	1 : 1 or 1 : 2	Invasive
III	Covering physician in hospital with resuscitation skills	1 : 3 or 1 : 4	Limited invasive
IV	Physician on call	1 : 3 to 1 : 5	Noninvasive

From NIH Consensus on ICU classification.

GRADING SYSTEM FOR MOTOR STRENGTH

GRADE	DESCRIPTION
0	No contraction
1	Flicker or trace of contraction, but unable to move extremity across a joint
2	Able to move extremity with gravity eliminated
3	Able to move against gravity, but with no resistance
4	Movement against some resistance
5	Normal strength

From Aids to the Examination of the Peripheral Nervous System. The Medical Research Council, 1986.

CLASSIFICATION OF ABDOMINAL TRAUMA BY ZONE

ZONE	LOCATION
I	This zone is the centromedial portion of the retroperitoneum. It contains the duodenum, pancreas, and all of the major abdominal blood vessels.
II	This zone is the area lateral to Zone I and includes both kidneys and the retroperitoneal colon.
III	This zone includes the entire pelvis.

In general, Zone I hematomas require exploration, because vascular injuries in this area can be quickly fatal. The treatment of Zone II injuries may involve surgery or observation alone, depending on the result of initial radiologic work-up and the patient's overall condition. Zone III hematomas frequently result from pelvic fractures and may require orthopedic stabilization rather than pelvic exploration.

From Ritchie WP, Steele G, Dean RH (eds): General Surgery. Philadelphia: J.B. Lippincott, 1995:888–893.

ZONES OF THE NECK

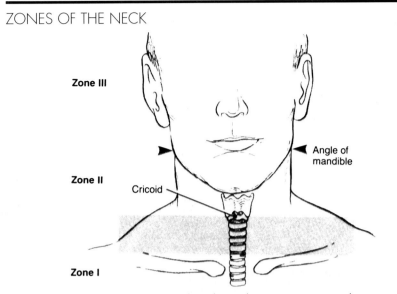

Zone I is the area beneath the clavicles, whereas Zone III is the area above the angle of the mandible. Penetrating Zone II trauma requires exploration in most cases if the platysma is penetrated. Injuries in either Zone I or III often are studied by noninvasive or invasive tests before surgery.

From Moore EE (ed): Early Care of the Injured Patient, 4th ed. Toronto: B.C. Decker, 1990:127.

MICROBIAL STAGING OF BURN WOUNDS

STAGE	DESCRIPTION
Ia	Superficial burn wound colonization
Ib	Penetrating burn wound colonization of the eschar
Ic	Dense population of microorganisms at the nonviable-viable tissue interface
IIa	Small foci of organisms in the most superficial viable tissue
IIb	Multifocal or generalized spread of microorganisms into viable tissue
IIc	Microorganisms present in small blood vessels and lymphatics

In general, tissues are said to be infected when $> 10^5$ organisms/cubic centimenter are present.

From Moylan JA: Principles of Trauma Surgery. New York: Gower Publishing, 1992:13.19.

CLASSIFICATION OF BURNS BY BODY SURFACE AREA ("THE RULE OF NINES")

The total percent of the body burned is calculated by using the following estimates:

18%	Front of the torso
18%	Back
18%	Each lower extremity
9%	Each upper extremity
9%	Head
1%	Perineum

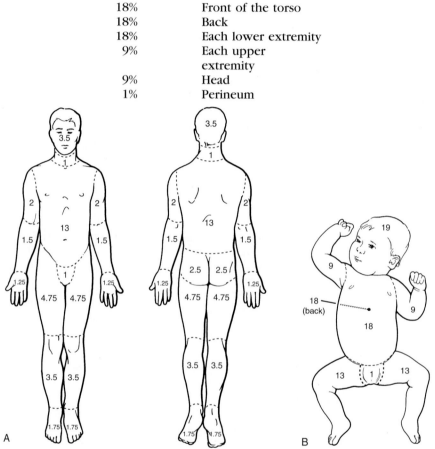

The above percentages are not applicable to children, and the anatomical charts are much more accurate both in adults and children. Also, remember that the palm—excluding the fingers—is considered to represent 1% of the total body surface area.

*From Marks MW, Marks C (eds): **Fundamentals of Plastic Surgery. Philadelphia: W.B. Saunders, 1997:51–52.***

BURN DEPTH
▷ Characteristics of First-, Second-, and Third-Degree Burns

	1st	**2nd**	**3rd**
Cause	Sunlight, minor flash	Scald, flash, chemicals	Flame, chemicals, electrical
Color	Light pink, slight darkening	Pink or mottled red	Pearly white, translucent; deep red in infants
Texture	Dry or small blisters	Blister or wet surface	Dry, thrombosed superficial vessels, spongy necrosis with alkali
Sensation	Painful	Painful	Anesthetic
Healing	3–6 days	10–21 days	Requires grafting

In clinical practice, it often is difficult to distinguish between first- and second-degree burns. It is perhaps more clinically helpful to classify burns as partial thickness (will heal) versus full thickness (require excision and grafting).

From Lopez-Viego M (ed): The Parkland Trauma Handbook. St. Louis: Mosby, 1994:392.

BURN DEPTH
▷ Characteristics of Partial and Full Thickness Burns

	PARTIAL	**FULL**
Cause	Hot liquids, flashes, dilute chemicals	Flame, high-voltage electricity, concentrated chemicals, hot metal
Color	Pink, mottled red	Pearly white or charred; translucent and parchment-like
Surface	Blisters, moist and weeping	Dry with shreds of nonviable epidermis, thrombosed vessels
Texture	Pliable	Inelastic and leathery
Sensation	Hypersensitive	Hypalgesic
Healing	10–35 days	Grafting required

Partial thickness burns may evolve into full thickness burns because of infection, ischemia, or poor wound care.

From Moylan JA: Principles of Trauma. New York: Gower Publishing, 1992:13.13.

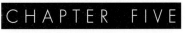

CHAPTER FIVE

Pediatric Surgery

STAGING OF NECROTIZING ENTEROCOLITIS

STAGE	CHARACTERISTICS
I (Suspected)	Any one or more historical factors that produce perinatal stress
	Systemic manifestations, including temperature instability, lethargy, apnea, bradycardia
	Gastrointestinal manifestations, including poor feeding, increasing pregavage residuals, emesis, mild abdominal distention, occult blood in stools
	Abdominal radiographs showing distention and mild ileus
II (Definite)	Any one or more historical factors
	Above signs and symptoms plus persistent occult or gross gastrointestinal bleeding and marked abdominal distention
	Abdominal radiographs showing significant intestinal distention with ileus, small bowel edema, pneumatosis intestinalis, and portal vein gas
III (Advanced)	Any one or more historical factors
	Above signs and symptoms plus deterioration of vital signs, evidence of septic shock, marked gastrointestinal hemorrhage
	Abdominal radiographs showing pneumoperitoneum in addition to findings listed for Stage II

Necrotizing enterocolitis is a spectrum of intraabdominal conditions that affects 1% to 2% of newborns, usually premature infants in a neonatal intensive care unit. The disease may be mild and self-limiting, or severe and life-threatening. The cause is usually unclear.

From Bell MJ, Kosloske A, Benton C, et al.: Neonatal necrotizing enterocolitis in infancy: Prevention of perforation. J Pediatr Surg 1973; 8:6013.

CLASSIFICATION OF THE MAJOR INTERSEX ABNORMALITIES

DIAGNOSIS	BUCCAL SMEAR	KARYOTYPE	URINARY STEROIDS	GONADS
Female pseudohermaphroditism	Positive	XX	Positive	Normal ovaries
True hermaphroditism	Positive	XX	Negative	Testis Ovary
Male pseudohermaphroditism	Negative	XY	Negative	Testes
Mixed gonadal dysgenesis	Negative	XO/XY	Negative	Streak ovaries

It is important to do genetic testing and careful physical examination prior to assigning a sex to these infants.

From Coran AG: The pediatric genitourinary system. In Greenfield L (ed): Surgery. Philadelphia: Lippincott Williams & Wilkins, 1993:1913.

TRACHEOESOPHAGEAL ("TE") FISTULA CLASSIFICATION

ESOPHAGEAL ATRESIA
TE FISTULA

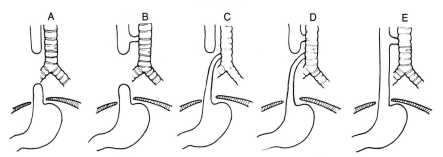

TYPE	DESCRIPTION
A	Proximal esophageal atresia without tracheal fistula (8%)
B	Proximal esophageal atresia with a proximal TE fistula (1%)
C	Proximal esophageal atresia with a distal TE fistula (85%)
D	Esophageal atresia with fistula between both proximal and distal ends of esophagus and trachea (2%)
E	Tracheoesophageal fistula without esophageal atresia, the so-called "H-type fistula" (4%)

The Type C TE fistula is by far the most common. The overall incidence of TE fistula is 1 in 1500 to 3000 births. Both sexes are equally affected. Ten percent of patients will have the VATER syndrome (vertebral, anorectal, tracheal, esophageal, renal, and radius anomalies).

From Sabiston DE (ed): Textbook of Surgery, 15th ed. Philadelphia: W.B. Saunders, 1997: 1237.

CLASSIFICATION OF JEJUNOILEAL ATRESIA

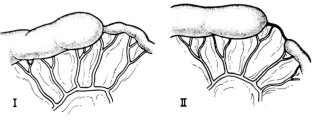

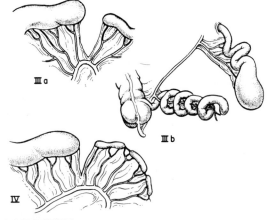

TYPE	DESCRIPTION
I	A mucosal web or diaphragm
II	Atretic cord exists between two blind ends of the bowel with an intact mesentary
IIIa	A complete separation of the blind ends of the bowel by a V-shaped mesentary gap defect
IIIb	Atresia with an apple-peel or Christmas tree deformity, in which the distal bowel receives a retrograde blood supply from the ileocolic or right colic artery
IV	Multiple atresias characterized by a "string of sausage" appearance

From Grosfeld JL, et al.: Operative management of intestinal atresia based on pathologic findings. J Pediatr Surg 1979; 14:368.

WINGSPREAD CLASSIFICATION OF ANORECTAL ANOMALIES

LEVEL	FEMALE	MALE
High	Anorectal agenesis with rectovaginal fistula	Anorectal agenesis with rectoprostatitis, urethral fistula
	Rectal atresia	Rectal atresia
Intermediate	Rectovestibular fistula	Rectobulbar urethral fistula
	Rectovaginal fistula	
	Anal agenesis without fistula	Anal agenesis without fistula
Low	Anovestibular fistula	Anocutaneous fistula
	Anocutaneous fistula	Anal stenosis
	Anal stenosis	Rare malformations
	Cloacal malformations	
	Rare malformations	

From Smith ED: The bath water needs changing but don't throw out the baby: An overview of anorectal anomalies. J Pediatr Surg 1988; 22:335.

RHABDOMYOSARCOMA STAGING
▷ Intergroup Rhabdomyosarcoma Study Group Staging System

STAGE	DESCRIPTION
1	Disease is found in the eye (orbit) or in the head, neck, or genitourinary areas. It has not spread to other areas of the body.
2	Tumor is not in the sites listed in Stage 1, is less than 5 cm in diameter, and has not spread to the lymph nodes.
3	Tumor is not in the sites listed in Stage 1, may be more than 5 cm in diameter, and may have spread to the lymph nodes near the tumor.
4	Disease has spread and is found in other parts of the body at the time of diagnosis (metastasis).

Rhabdomyosarcoma is a sarcoma that is diagnosed in about 250 American children each year. It is the most common soft tissue tumor in children and can occur in any body area. Treatment is a combination of radiation therapy, chemotherapy and surgery that is guided by stage of disease and one of the standard cancer treatment protocols.

From the Intergroup Rhabdomyosarcoma Study Group, http://rhabdo.org/rhabdo/stagrhab.htm.

WILMS' TUMOR (NEPHROBLASTOMA) STAGING

STAGE	DESCRIPTION
I	Tumor limited to the kidney and completely resected
II	Tumor extends beyond the kidney but is completely resected; capsule invasion, perirenal tissues may be involved
III	Residual nonhematogenous tumor confined to the abdomen, including tumor rupture or peritoneal implants; lymph nodes involved, present after nephrectomy
IV	Hematogenous metastases (lung, brain, distant lymph nodes)
V	Bilateral renal involvement at diagnosis

Of the 500 new cases detected each year, most occur in children aged 1 to 4 years. These patients should be managed according to the most recent protocols from the National Wilms' Tumor Study Group.

From Sabiston DE: Textbook of Surgery, 14th ed. Philadelphia: W.B. Saunders, 1991:1179.

CLASSIFICATION OF PREMATURE INFANTS VERSUS SMALL FOR GESTATIONAL AGE (SGA) INFANTS

CHARACTERISTIC	SGA INFANTS	PREMATURE INFANTS
Fetal demise	+++	+
Neonatal demise	++	+++
Congenital malformation	+++	+/−
Weight changes	<5% loss, then 5%–10% rapid gain	loss then slow gain
Hyaline membrane disease	+	+++
Meconium aspiration	+++	+
Apnea	+	+++
Hypothermia	++++	++
Hyperbilirubinemia	+	++++
Hematocrit	Normal/high	Normal/low
Intracranial hemorrhage	+	+++
Necrotizing enterocolitis	+	+++
Persistent fetal circulation	++	+

From Rowe M, Tagge EP: Pediatric physiology. In Greenfield L (ed): Surgery. Philadelphia: Lippincott Williams & Wilkins, 1993:1792.

NEUROBLASTOMA STAGING
▷ Evans Staging System

STAGE	DESCRIPTION
I	Tumor confined to organ of origin (totally excised)
II	Tumor extends beyond organ of origin but does not cross the midline; regional lymph nodes may be involved
III	Tumor extends beyond the midline to encroach on tissues on opposite side
IV	Distant metastasis (skeletal, other solid organs, soft tissues, distant lymph nodes)
V(IV S)	Localized primary tumor not crossing midline with remote disease confined to liver, subcutaneous tissues, and bone marrow, but without evidence of bone cortex involvement

*From Evans AE, D'Angio GJ, Randolph JG: **A proposed staging system for children with neuroblastoma. Cancer 1971; 27:374.***

▷ International Staging System

STAGE	DESCRIPTION
I	Localized tumor confined to the area of origin; complete gross excision, with or without microscopic residual disease; identifiable ipsilateral and contralateral lymph nodes negative microscopically
IIA	Unilateral tumor with incomplete gross excision; identifiable ipsilateral and contralateral lymph nodes negative microscopically
IIB	Unilateral tumor with complete or incomplete gross excision; with positive ipsilateral lymph nodes; identifiable contralateral lymph nodes negative microscopically
III	Tumor infiltrating across the midline with or without regional lymph node involvement; or unilateral tumor with contralateral regional lymph node involvement; or midline tumor with bilateral regional lymph node involvement
IV	Dissemination of tumor to distant lymph nodes, bone, bone marrow, liver, and/or other organs
IV S	Localized primary tumor as defined for Stage I or IIA, with dissemination limited to liver, skin, or bone marrow

Two key determinants of survival are age of patient and stage. Stage IV S has an 80% survival and is a better prognosis than Stage II, III, or IV.

*From Smith EL, et al.: **Surgical perspective on the current staging in neuroblastoma: The International Neuroblastoma Staging System Proposal. J Pediatr Surg 1989; 24:386.***

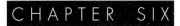

CHAPTER SIX

Plastic Surgery

SCHOBINGER STAGING SYSTEM OF ARTERIOVENOUS MALFORMATIONS

STAGE	DESCRIPTION
I	Blush/stain, warmth, and arteriovenous shunting by continuous Doppler or 20-MHz color Doppler
II	Same as Stage I, plus enlargement, tortuous tense veins, pulsations, thrill, and bruit
III	Same as above, plus either dystrophic changes, ulceration, bleeding, persistent pain, or destruction
IV	Same as Stage II, plus cardiac failure

Arteriovenous malformations are fast-flow lesions, and the clinical diagnosis is confirmed by ultrasonography and color Doppler study. Schobinger Stage III and IV lesions usually require some type of definitive treatment.

From Aston SJ, Beasley RW, Thorne CHM (eds): Grabb and Smith's Plastic Surgery, 5th ed. Philadelphia: Lippincott-Raven, 1997:201.

CLASSIFICATION OF MELANOMA BY DEPTH—BRESLOW'S LEVELS

STAGE	THICKNESS	PROGNOSIS
1	0-0.75 mm	Best
2	0.76-1.50 mm	Intermediate
3	1.51-3.0 mm	Intermediate
4	>3.0 mm	Worst, high chance of metastases

The Breslow staging technique uses an oculomicrometer to measure the actual maximum depth of penetration by the tumor. The depth of tumor penetration should be indicated on the pathology report. The above thickness ranges are only a crude means of grouping tumors by relative thickness and eventual prognosis.

From Breslow A: Thickness, cross-sectional areas and depth of invasion in the prognosis of cutaneous melanoma. Ann Surg 1970; 172:902.

CLASSIFICATION OF MELANOMA BY DEPTH—CLARK'S LEVELS

LEVEL	DESCRIPTION
1	Intraepidermal: cells superficial to the basement membrane
2	Papillary dermal: cells extend through the basement membrane to papillary dermis
3	Papillary—reticular interface: cells begin to accumulate at the interface between papillary and reticular dermis
4	Reticular dermal: cells extend between bundles of reticular dermis collagen
5	Invasion of subcutaneous tissue

Clark levels of invasion predict survival, because deeper tumors have a worse prognosis. The Clark levels, however, vary from one region of the body to another as the dermal elements vary in thickness from one part to another. For this reason, the Breslow levels may be a more accurate and consistent classification system.

Text from Clark WH Jr: A classification of malignant melanoma in man correlated with histogenesis and biologic behavior. In Montagana W, Hu F (eds): Advances in Biology of the Skin. London: Pergamon Press, 1967:621. Illustration from Marks MW, Marks C (eds): Fundamentals of Plastic Surgery. Philadelphia: W.B. Saunders, 1997:38.

CLASSIFICATION OF NECK TYPES

CLASS	DESCRIPTION
I	Well-defined mentocervical angle, with good skin and muscle tone
II	Ptosis of the cervical soft tissues, with little fat accumulation and normal platysma tone
III	Submental fat accumulation, either congenital or acquired
IV	Platysmal banding on repose or contraction
V	Retrognathia or microgenia present
VI	Low-positioned hyoid bone, with a poorly defined mentocervical angle

From Dedo DD: A preoperative classification of the neck for cervicofacial rhytidectomy. Laryngoscope 1980; 90:984–986.

NUMBERING OF TEETH
▷ Universal System (Most common)

PERMANENT TEETH
The maxillary teeth are numbered 1 to 16 from right to left, and the mandibular teeth are numbered 17 to 32 from left to right.

Right	1	2	3	4	5	6	7	8	9	10	11	12	13	14	15	16	Left
	32	31	30	29	28	27	26	25	24	23	22	21	20	19	18	17	

PRIMARY TEETH
The 20 primary (deciduous) teeth are described by letters, with the maxillary teeth labelled A to J from right to left, and the mandibular teeth labelled K to T from left to right.

Right	A	B	C	D	E	F	G	H	I	J	Left
	T	S	R	Q	P	O	N	M	L	K	

▷ Palmer System (Used by American orthodontists)

Right	8	7	6	5	4	3	2	1	1	2	3	4	5	6	7	8	Left
	8	7	6	5	4	3	2	1	1	2	3	4	5	6	7	8	

PERMANENT TEETH
The teeth are numbered from 1 to 8 in each of the four quadrants, starting with the central incisor (1) and ending with the third molar (8). The quadrant is indicated by a bracket around the number.

▷ ISO/FDI SYSTEM

PERMANENT TEETH

Right	18	17	16	15	14	13	12	11	21	22	23	24	25	26	27	28	Left
	48	47	46	45	44	43	42	41	31	32	33	34	35	36	37	38	

DECIDUOUS TEETH

Right	55	54	53	52	51	61	62	63	64	65	Left
	85	84	83	82	81	71	72	73	74	75	

PERMANENT TEETH
Each tooth is assigned a two-digit number where the first number is the quadrant number (1 to 4) and the second is the tooth number as in the Palmer system. Therefore, the mandibular left central incisor would be "three-one."

PRIMARY TEETH
The quadrants are 5 to 8 and the teeth are 1 to 5 from central incisor to second molar. Therefore, the mandibular left central incisor would be "seven-one."

From Weinzweig J: **Plastic Surgery Secrets. Philadelphia: Hanley & Belfus, 1999:123–124.**

BAKER CLASSIFICATION OF BREAST IMPLANT CAPSULAR CONTRACTURE

Grade I	Soft
Grade II	Minimal contracture; implant palpable but not visible
Grade III	Moderate contracture; implant palpable and discernible
Grade IV	Severe contracture; hard symptomatic breast, sometimes with distortion

The rate of severe capsular contracture has fallen with the increased use of saline-filled implants. The rate of severe contracture at present is about 5%.

From Baker JL Jr: Classification of spherical contractures: Augmentation mammoplasty. In Owsley JQ Jr, Peterson RA (eds): Symposium on Aesthetic Surgery of the Breast. St. Louis: CV Mosby, 1978:256–263.

REGNAULT CLASSIFICATION OF BREAST PTOSIS

DEGREE	DESCRIPTION
1st	Location of the nipple-areola at or slightly above the inframammary fold (IMF) and above the lower convexity of the breast (Figure A)
2nd	The nipple-areola is below the IMF, but is situated on the anterior aspect of the breast mound (Figure B)
3rd	The nipple-areola is below the IMF and also on the dependent part of the inferior convexity of the breast (Figure C)

In pseudoptosis, the nipple-areola is actually above the IMF but the breast mound has descended below the IMF (Figure D).

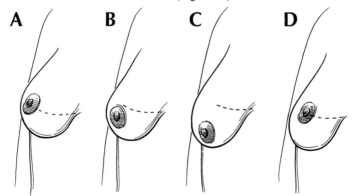

A   B   C   D

Text from Regnault P: Breast ptosis. Clin Plast Surg 1976; 3:193. Illustration from Marks MW, Marks C (eds): Fundamentals of Plastic Surgery. Philadelphia: W.B. Saunders, 1997:290.

TESSIER CLASSIFICATION OF CRANIOFACIAL CLEFTS

The 0 to 7 clefts represent facial clefts, whereas the 8 to 14 clefts represent the cranial extensions. A cleft of both the face and cranium can be described by two numbers (i.e., 3-11 cleft).
The bilateral combination of no. 6, 7, and 8 clefts is found in the Treacher Collins syndrome, and a no. 7 cleft alone is referred to as hemifacial microsomia.
Multiple and bilateral clefts can occur simultaneously.

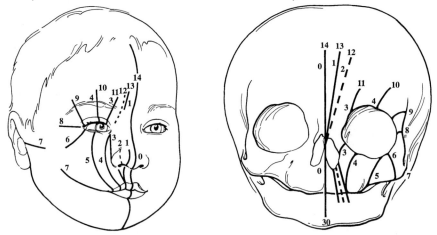

From Marks MW, Marks C (eds): **Fundamentals of Plastic Surgery.** *Philadelphia: W.B. Saunders, 1997:137.*

PRESSURE SORE STAGING

STAGE I—Nonblanchable erythema of intact skin.
STAGE II—Partial thickness skin loss involving epidermis, dermis, or both. Clinically, it appears as an abrasion, blister, or shallow crater.
STAGE III—Full-thickness skin loss involving damage or necrosis of subcutaneous tissue that may extend down to, but not through, underlying fascia. Clinically, there is a deep crater.
STAGE IV—Extensive destruction, tissue necrosis, or damage to muscle, bone, or supporting structures.

From Treatment of Pressure Ulcers Guideline Panel: **Treatment of Pressure Ulcers (Clinical Practice Guideline No. 15) U.S. Department of Health and Human Services/Public Health Service, 1994.**

CLASSIFICATION OF ORBITAL HYPERTELORISM

▷ Tessier System

TYPE	INTERORBITAL DISTANCE
I	30–34 mm
II	35–39 mm
III	>40 mm

The interorbital distance is the distance between the medial walls of the orbits at the junction of the frontal and lacrimal bones and the maxilla (the dacryon). Normal interorbital distance in men is 28 mm; in women, 25 mm.

From Tessier P, Tulasne JF: *Stability in correction of hypertelorbitism and Treacher Collins syndromes. Clin Plast Surg 1989; 16:195–199.*

▷ Munro System

TYPE	SHAPE OF MEDIAL ORBITAL WALLS
A	Parallel
B	Anterior portion balloons out
C	Central portion balloons out
D	Posterior portion balloons out

From Munro IR, Das SK: *Improving results in orbital hypertelorism correction. Ann Plast Surg 1979; 2:499–507.*

CLASSIFICATION OF CLEFT LIP AND PALATE

Cleft lip and palate deformities are best classified according to the anatomic structures that are involved. The primary palate is the lip, premaxilla, and alveolus. The secondary palate includes the hard and soft palate posterior to the incisive foramen.

CLEFT OF PRIMARY PALATE (CLEFT LIP)
Unilateral
    Incomplete—involves the lip only
    Complete—involves all structures of the primary palate
Bilateral
    Incomplete—involves the lip only
    Complete—involves all structures of the primary palate

CLEFT OF THE SECONDARY PALATE
Incomplete—involves the soft palate or the soft and part of the hard palate
Complete—involves the entire soft palate and the hard palate to the incisive foramen

COMBINATIONS OF CLEFTS
Combinations of the above clefting patterns frequently occur.

From Marks MW, Marks C (eds): **Fundamentals of Plastic Surgery.** *Philadelphia: W.B. Saunders, 1997:155–157.*

CLASSIFICATION OF NASO-ORBITAL-ETHMOID FRACTURES

TYPE	DESCRIPTION
I	The canthal ligament is attached to a *single* large medial fragment. This fracture may be either complete or incomplete.
II	The central fragment is comminuted, but the canthal ligament is attached to a fragment that can be stabilized with wires or plates.
III	There is severe comminution such that canthal detachment and reattachment is required to achieve adequate reduction.

All of these types may be either unilateral or bilateral.

From Markowitz BL, Manson PN, Sargent L, et al.: **Management of the medial canthal tendon in nasoethmoidal fractures: The importance of the central fragment in classification and treatment. Plast Reconstr Surg 1991; 87:843–853.**

ANGLE'S CLASSIFICATION OF OCCLUSION

The reference point is the upper first molar. In Class I occlusion, the maxillary first molar mesiobuccal cusp is aligned with the mandibular first molar mesiobuccal groove. In Class II occlusion, the maxillary mesiobuccal cusp is anterior to the mesiobuccal groove of the mandibular first molar. In Class III occlusion, the mesiobuccal cusp sits posterior to the mesiobuccal groove of the mandibular first molar.

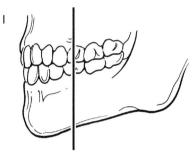

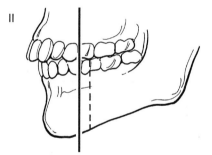

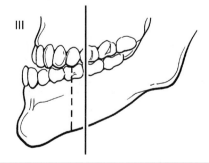

From Marks MW, Marks C (eds): **Fundamentals of Plastic Surgery. Philadelphia: W.B. Saunders, 1997:148.**

KNIGHT AND NORTH CLASSIFICATION OF ZYGOMA FRACTURES

GROUP	DESCRIPTION
I	Undisplaced
II	Displaced arch
III	Depressed body without rotation
IV	Depressed with medial rotation
V	Depressed with lateral rotation
VI	Complex

From Knight JS, North JF: The classification of malar fractures: An analysis of displacement as a guide to treatment. Br J Plast Surg 1960; 13:325–339.

CRANIOSYNOSTOSIS CLASSIFICATION

SUTURE AFFECTED	DEFORMITY
Metopic suture	Trigoncephaly
Sagittal suture	Scaphocephaly
Unilateral coronal suture	Frontal plagiocephaly
Bilateral coronal sutures	Frontal brachycephaly
Sagittal and both coronals	Oxycephaly
Unilateral lambdoid	Occipital plagiocephaly
Bilateral lambdoid	Occipital brachycephaly

From Marks MW, Marks C (eds): Fundamentals of Plastic Surgery. Philadelphia: W.B. Saunders, 1997:141.

MATHES AND NAHAI CLASSIFICATION OF MUSCLE FLAP BLOOD SUPPLY

TYPE I—The muscle's major blood supply is from a single dominant pedicle (examples: gastrocnemius and tensor fasciae latae).
TYPE II—There is a dual blood supply with a dominant and a minor blood supply (examples: gracilis, soleus, trapezius).
TYPE III—The muscle has two major pedicles (example: rectus abdominis).
TYPE IV—The muscle has multiple pedicles (example: sartorius).
TYPE V—The muscle has one major blood supply and a number of secondary pedicles (examples: latissimus dorsi and pectoralis major).

From Mathes SJ, Nahai F: Clinical Applications for Muscle and Musculocutaneous Flaps. St. Louis: Mosby Year Book, 1982.

GLOGAU'S CLASSIFICATION OF PHOTOAGING GROUPS

GROUP	DESCRIPTION
I (mild)	Usually 28–35 yrs No keratoses, little wrinkling, no acne scarring Little or no makeup
II (moderate)	Usually 35–50 yrs Early actinic keratoses—subtle skin yellowing Early wrinkling—parallel smile lines Mild acne scarring Little makeup
III (advanced)	Usually 50–65 yrs Actinic keratoses—obvious skin yellowing with telangiectasia Wrinkling—present at rest Moderate acne scarring Wears makeup always
IV (severe)	Usually 65–75 yrs Actinic keratoses and skin cancer have occurred Wrinkling—much cutis laxa Severe acne scarring Wears makeup that does not cover but cakes on

Most patients with sun-damaged skin fall into one of these general categories.

From Brody HJ: **Chemical Peeling.** *St. Louis: Mosby, 1992:38.*

FITZPATRICK'S CLASSIFICATION OF SUN-REACTIVE SKIN TYPES

TYPE	COLOR	REACTION TO FIRST SUMMER EXPOSURE
I	White	Always burn, never tan
II	White	Usually burn, tan with difficulty
III	White	Sometimes mild burn, tan average
IV	Moderate brown	Rarely burn, tan with ease
V	Dark brown	Very rarely burn, tan very easily
VI	Black	Never burn, tan very easily

From Brody HJ: **Chemical Peeling.** *St. Louis: Mosby, 1992:36.*

NORWOOD CLASSIFICATION OF MALE PATTERN BALDNESS

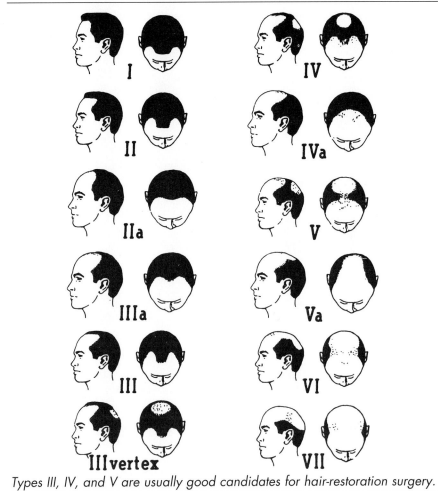

Types III, IV, and V are usually good candidates for hair-restoration surgery.

From Hordinsky: *Atlas of Hair and Nails*. Philadelphia: Churchill Livingstone, 2000.

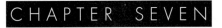

CHAPTER SEVEN

Orthopedic and Hand Surgery

PELVIC FRACTURE CLASSIFICATION
▷ (Young and Resnik's modification of the Pennel and Tile Classification)

ANTEROPOSTERIOR COMPRESSION

Type I — Disruption of the pubic symphysis with less than 2.5 cm of diastasis; no significant posterior pelvic injury ("open book injury"). *Stable.*

Type II — Disruption of the pubic symphysis of more than 2.5 cm with tearing of the anterior sacroiliac, sacrospinous, and sacrotuberous ligaments. *Rotationally unstable.*

Type III — Complete disruption of the pubic symphysis and posterior ligament complexes, with hemipelvic displacement.

LATERAL COMPRESSION

Type I — Posterior compression of the sacroiliac joint without ligament disruption; oblique pubic ramus fracture. *Stable.*

Type II — Rupture of the posterior sacroiliac ligament; pivotal internal rotation of hemipelvis on the anterior S1 joint with a crush injury of the sacrum and an oblique pubic ramus fracture.

Type III — Findings in Type II injury with evidence of an anteroposterior compression injury to the contralateral hemipelvis.

VERTICAL SHEAR

Complete ligament or bony disruption of a hemipelvis associated with hemipelvis displacement.

Pelvic fractures can be simple with little blood loss, or severe with life-threatening arterial hemorrhage. This grading system ranks pelvic fractures in increasing likelihood of major bleeding and other severe injuries. Anteroposterior injuries frequently are seen in pedestrians and motorcyclists, whereas lateral compression injuries often result from motor vehicle accidents. Vertical shear injuries often result from falls.

Young JW, Resnick CS: Fracture of the pelvis: Current concepts of classification. AJR 1990; 155:1169.

CLASSIFICATION OF OPEN FRACTURES
TYPE   **DESCRIPTION**

I   Skin opening of 1 cm or less, quite clean. Minimal muscle contusion. Simple transverse or short oblique fractures.
II   Lacerations more than 1 cm long, with extensive soft tissue damage, flaps, or avulsion. Minimal to moderate crushing component. Simple transverse or short oblique fractures with minimal comminution.
III   Extensive soft tissue damage, including muscles, skin, and neurovascular structures. Often a high-velocity injury with severe crushing component.
IIIA   Extensive soft tissue laceration, adequate bone coverage. Segmental fractures, gunshot injuries.
IIIB   Extensive soft tissue injury with periosteal stripping and bone exposure. Usually associated with massive contamination.
IIIC   Vascular injury requiring repair.

From Gustilo RB, et al.: Problems in the management of type III (severe) open fractures: A new classification of type III open fractures. J Trauma 1984; 24:742–746.

MASON CLASSIFICATION OF RADIAL HEAD AND NECK FRACTURES
TYPE   **DESCRIPTION**

I   Undisplaced segmental (marginal) fracture
II   Displaced segmental fracture
III   Comminuted fracture
IV   Type III associated with posterior dislocation of the elbow

From Morrey BF: The Elbow and Its Disorders. Philadelphia: W.B. Saunders, 1985. Copyright Mayo Clinic.

CLASSIFICATION OF HANGMAN'S FRACTURES

TYPE	DESCRIPTION
I	Fracture through the pars region of C1 without displacement
II	Fracture through the pars region of C1 with a ligamentous injury to the disc complex, allowing displacement of the body by more than 3 mm
III	Fracture through the pars region with dislocation of the C2 and C3 facets

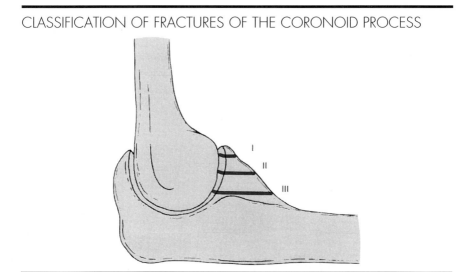

Type I   Type II   Type III

From Browner B, Jupiter JB, Levine AM, Trafton PG (eds): Skeletal Trauma, 2nd ed. Philadelphia: W.B. Saunders, 1998:821.

CLASSIFICATION OF FRACTURES OF THE CORONOID PROCESS

From Regan W, Morrey B: Fractures of the coronoid process of the ulna. J Bone Joint Surg 1989; 71A:1348.

DELLON MODIFICATION OF HIGHET'S CLASSIFICATION OF NERVE REPAIR OUTCOME

STAGE	DESCRIPTION
MOTOR	
M0	No contraction
M1	Return of perceptible contraction in the proximal muscles
M2	Return of perceptible contraction in the proximal and distal muscles
M3	Return of function in both proximal and distal muscles of such a degree that all important muscles are sufficiently powerful to act against gravity
M4	M3 plus all synergistic and independent movements are possible
M5	Complete recovery
SENSORY	
S0	Absence of sensibility in the autonomous area
S1	Recovery of deep cutaneous pain sensibility within the autonomous area of the nerve
S2	Return of some degree of superficial cutaneous pain and tactile sensibility within the autonomous area of the nerve
S3	Return of superficial cutaneous pain and tactile sensibility throughout the autonomous area, with disappearance of any previous overresponse
S3+	S3 plus recovery of some two-point discrimination within the autonomous area (7–15 mm)
S4	Complete recovery (two-point discrimination, 2–6 mm)

From Dellon AL, Curtis RM, Edgerton MT: Reeducation of sensation in the hand after nerve injury and repair. Plast Reconstruct Surg 1974; 53:297–305.

CLASSIFICATION OF DISTAL HUMERAL INTERCONDYLAR FRACTURES

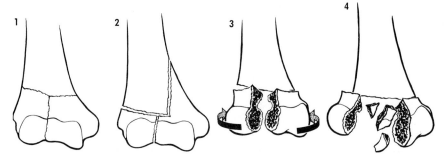

Type 2 and 3 fractures usually are treated by open reduction and internal fixation (ORIF). Type 4 fractures most often are treated without surgery unless reconstruction is thought to be technically possible.

From Rockwood CA, Green DP (eds): Fractures in Adults, 2nd ed. Philadelphia: J.B. Lippincott, 1984.

HERBERT CLASSIFICATION OF SCAPHOID FRACTURES

TYPE A:
STABLE ACUTE FRACTURES

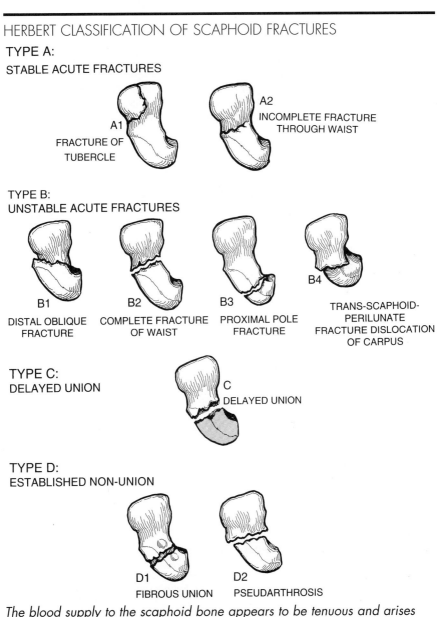

A1
FRACTURE OF
TUBERCLE

A2
INCOMPLETE FRACTURE
THROUGH WAIST

TYPE B:
UNSTABLE ACUTE FRACTURES

B1
DISTAL OBLIQUE
FRACTURE

B2
COMPLETE FRACTURE
OF WAIST

B3
PROXIMAL POLE
FRACTURE

B4
TRANS-SCAPHOID-
PERILUNATE
FRACTURE DISLOCATION
OF CARPUS

TYPE C:
DELAYED UNION

C
DELAYED UNION

TYPE D:
ESTABLISHED NON-UNION

D1
FIBROUS UNION

D2
PSEUDARTHROSIS

The blood supply to the scaphoid bone appears to be tenuous and arises distally, so that the fractured proximal part is at risk for avascular necrosis and eventual non-union.

From Herbert TJ: The Fractured Scaphoid. St. Louis: Quality Medical Publishing, 1990:52.

ANDERSON AND D'ALONZO'S CLASSIFICATION OF ODONTOID FRACTURES

TYPE	DESCRIPTION
I	Fractures of the tip of the odontoid process
II	Fractures that penetrate the base of the odontoid
III	Fractures that extend into the body of C2

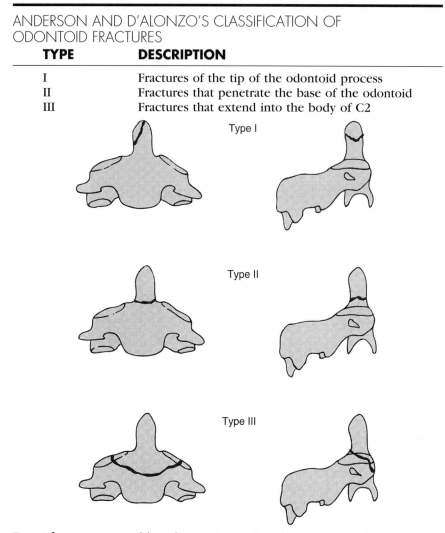

Type I

Type II

Type III

Type I fractures are stable, whereas Types II and III are not and require some form of stabilization.

From Anderson LD, D'Alonzo RT: Fractures of the odontoid process of the axis. J Bone Joint Surg 1974; 56A:1664.

WINQUIST-HANSEN CLASSIFICATION OF COMMINUTION

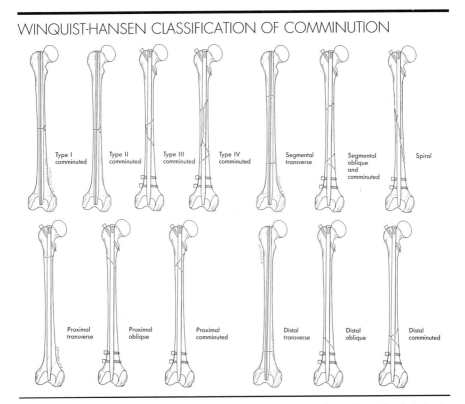

Illustration from Canale ST (ed): Campbell's Operative Orthopedics, 9th ed. St. Louis: Mosby, 1998:2142. Scheme from Winquist RA, Hansen RT, Clawson DK: Closed intramedullary nailing of femoral fractures: A report of 520 cases. J Bone Joint Surg 1984; 66A:529.

WASSEL CLASSIFICATION OF THUMB DUPLICATION

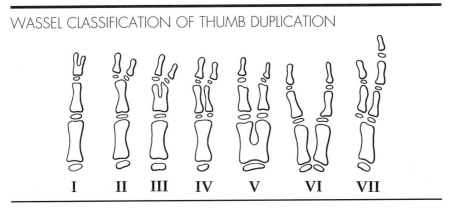

Illustration from Marks MW, Marks C (eds): Fundamentals of Plastic Surgery. Philadelphia: W.B. Saunders, 1997:384. Scheme from Wassel HD: Results of surgery for polydactyly of the thumb. Clin Orthop 1969; 64:175–193.

HOUSE CLASSIFICATION OF HAND FUNCTION

CLASS	DESIGNATION	ACTIVITY LEVEL
0	Does not use	Does not use
1	Poor passive assist	Uses as a stabilizing weight only
2	Fair passive assist	Can hold on to object placed in hand
3	Good passive assist	Can hold object and stabilize for use by other hand
4	Poor active assist	Can actively grasp object and hold it weakly
5	Fair active assist	Can actively grasp object and stabilize it well
6	Good active assist	Can actively grasp object and stabilize it well and manipulate object against other hand
7	Spontaneous use, partial	Can perform bimanual activities easily; occasionally uses the hand spontaneously
8	Spontaneous use, complete	Uses hand completely independently, without reference to the other hand

This classification system is used mainly in cerebral palsy patients to determine small improvements in hand function, but may be used in other patients as well.

From House JH, Gwathmey FW, Fidler MO: A dynamic approach to the thumb-in-palm deformity in cerebral palsy. Evaluation and results in 56 patients. J Bone Joint Surg 1981; 63A:216–225.

CLASSIFICATION OF PATELLAR FRACTURES

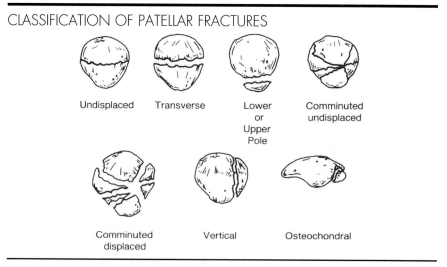

Undisplaced   Transverse   Lower or Upper Pole   Comminuted undisplaced

Comminuted displaced   Vertical   Osteochondral

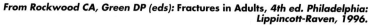
From Rockwood CA, Green DP (eds): Fractures in Adults, 4th ed. Philadelphia: Lippincott-Raven, 1996.

CLASSIFICATION OF PEDIATRIC FRACTURES OF THE PROXIMAL RADIUS

TYPE		DESCRIPTION
I		Valgus fractures
	A	Salter-Harris Types I and II
	B	Salter-Harris Type IV
	C	Fracture of the radial metaphysis only
II		Fractures secondary to posterior elbow dislocation
	D	Reduction injuries
	E	Dislocation injuries

From Rockwood CA (ed): Fractures in Children. Philadelphia: J.B. Lippincott, 1984.

CLASSIFICATION OF ACROMIOCLAVICULAR INJURIES

TYPE	DESCRIPTION
I	Neither acromioclavicular nor coracoclavicular ligaments are disrupted
II	Acromioclavicular ligament is disrupted, but coracoclavicular ligament is intact
III	Both ligaments are disrupted
IV	Ligaments are disrupted, and distal end of clavicle is displaced posteriorly into or through trapezius muscle
V	Ligaments and muscle attachments are disrupted, and clavicle and acromion are widely separated
VI	Ligaments are disrupted, and distal clavicle is dislocated inferior to coracoid process and posterior to biceps and coracobrachialis tendons

From Rockwood CA, Green DP (eds): Fractures in Adults, 2nd ed. Philadelphia: J.B. Lippincott, 1984.

NEER-HORWITZ CLASSIFICATION OF PEDIATRIC PROXIMAL HUMERAL FRACTURES

GRADE	DISPLACEMENT
I	<5 mm
II	$<1/3$ shaft width
III	2/3 shaft width
IV	$>2/3$ shaft width

From Neer CS, Horwitz BS: Fractures of the proximal humeral epiphyseal plate. Clin Orthop 1965; 41:24.

LAUGE-HANSEN CLASSIFICATION OF ANKLE FRACTURES

SUPINATION-ADDUCTION (SA)
1. Transverse avulsion-type fracture of the fibula below the level of the joint or tear of the lateral collateral ligaments
2. Vertical fracture of the medial malleolus

SUPINATION-EVERSION (SER—EXTERNAL ROTATION)
1. Disruption of the anterior tibiofibular ligament
2. Spiral oblique fracture of the distal fibula
3. Disruption of the posterior tibiofibular ligament or fracture of the posterior malleolus
4. Fracture of the medial malleolus or rupture of the deltoid ligament

PRONATION-ABDUCTION (PA)
1. Transverse fracture of the medial malleolus or rupture of the deltoid ligament
2. Rupture of the syndesmotic ligaments or avulsion fracture of their insertion(s)
3. Short, horizontal, oblique fracture of the fibula above the level of the joint

PRONATION-EVERSION (PER—EXTERNAL ROTATION)
1. Transverse fracture of the medial malleolus or disruption of the deltoid ligament
2. Disruption of the anterior tibiofibular ligament
3. Short oblique fracture of the fibula above the level of the joint
4. Rupture of the posterior tibiofibular ligament or avulsion fracture of the posterolateral tibia

PRONATION-DORSIFLEXION (PD)
1. Fracture of the medial malleolus
2. Fracture of the anterior margin of the tibia
3. Supramalleolar fracture of the fibula
4. Transverse fracture of the posterior tibial surface

The first word of the primary designations refers to the foot's position at the time of fracture, whereas the second word refers to the direction of the deforming force.

The most common mechanism of injury is supination-external rotation, and this results in a spiral oblique fracture of the distal fibula and rupture of the deltoid ligaments or fracture of the medial malleolus.

From Rockwood CA, Green DP (eds): Fractures in Adults, 4th ed. Philadelphia: Lippincott-Raven, 1996.

SCHATZKER CLASSIFICATION OF TIBIAL PLATEAU FRACTURES

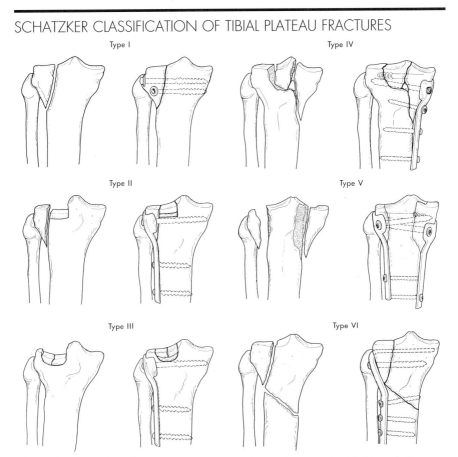

Type I

Type IV

Type II

Type V

Type III

Type VI

The Schatzker classification system is similar to the one by Hohl and Moore but adds type VI, metaphyseal-diaphyseal dissociation.

Illustration from Canale ST (ed): Campbell's Operative Orthopedics, 9th ed. St. Louis: Mosby, 1998:2097. Scheme from Schatzker J, McBroom R, Bruce D: The tibial plateau fracture: The Toronto experience 1968-1975. Clin Orthop 1979; 138:94.

ROCKWOOD AND DAMERON CLASSIFICATION OF PEDIATRIC DISTAL CLAVICLE FRACTURES

TYPE	DESCRIPTION
I	No displacement
II	A displaced fracture, but nonarticular
III	A fracture involving the acromioclavicular joint

From Green NE, Swintkowski MF (eds): Skeletal Trauma in Children, 2nd ed. Philadelphia: W.B. Saunders, 1998:323.

AO CLASSIFICATION OF MALLEOLAR FRACTURES

TYPE		DESCRIPTION
A		Fibula fracture below syndesmosis (*infrasyndesmotic*)
	A1	Isolated
	A2	With fracture of medial malleolus
	A3	With a posteromedial fracture
B		Fibula fracture at level of syndesmosis (*transsyndesmotic*)
	B1	Isolated
	B2	With a medial lesion (malleolus or ligament)
	B3	With a medial lesion and fracture of posterolateral tibia
C		Fibula fracture above syndesmosis (*suprasyndesmotic*)
	C1	Diaphyseal fracture of the fibula, simple
	C2	Diaphyseal fracture of the fibula, complex
	C3	Proximal fracture of the fibula

From Rockwood CA, Green DP (eds): Fractures in Adults, 4th ed. Philadelphia: Lippincott-Raven, 1996.

GERTZBEIN COMPREHENSIVE CLASSIFICATION OF SPINE INJURIES

TYPE		DESCRIPTION
A		Vertebral body compression fractures
	A1	Impaction injuries, mostly wedge fractures
	A2	Split fractures; pincer fracture most common
	A3	Burst fractures
B		Anterior and posterior element injury with distraction
	B1	Flexion-distraction injuries resulting in disruption of soft tissues posteriorly through the capsule of the facet joints
	B2	Flexion-distraction injuries resulting in disruption of soft tissues posteriorly through the bony arch
	B3	Anterior disruption through the disc, with or without associated fractures or soft tissue injuries of the posterior elements
C		Anterior and posterior element injury with rotation
	C1	Rotation associated with compression
	C2	Rotation associated with distraction
	C3	Rotation associated with rotational shear

Type A fractures are the most stable and have the least amount of bone and soft tissue disruption, and Type C are the most unstable and have the most tissue disruption.

From Gertzbein SD (ed): Fractures of the Thoracic and Lumbar Spine. Baltimore: Williams & Wilkins, 1992.

DELBET CLASSIFICATION OF PEDIATRIC PROXIMAL FEMUR FRACTURES

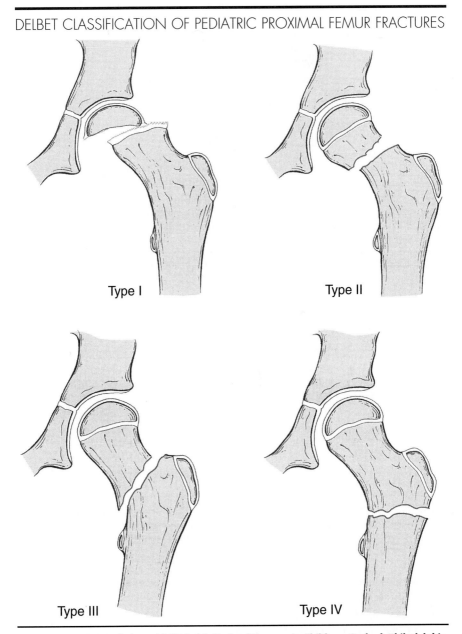

Type I

Type II

Type III

Type IV

*From Green NE, Swintkowski MF (eds): **Skeletal Trauma in Children, 2nd ed. Philadelphia: W.B. Saunders, 1998:390.***

CLASSIFICATION OF ACUTE DORSAL PROXIMAL INTERPHALANGEAL JOINT DISLOCATIONS

TYPE	DESCRIPTION
I	*Hyperextension*—the volar plate is avulsed and an incomplete longitudinal split occurs in the collateral ligaments. The articular surfaces remain in contact.
II	*Dorsal dislocation*—there is complete rupture of the volar plate and a complete split in the collateral ligaments. The proximal and middle phalanges are in an almost parallel alignment.
III	*Fracture dislocation*—the insertion of the volar plate, including a portion of the volar base of the middle phalanx, is disrupted. A major articular defect may be present.

Type I and II dislocations usually are stable once reduced and need protection for several days. Type III injuries, when unstable, usually require operative fixation.

From Eaton RG, Little JW: Joint injuries and their sequelae. Clin Plast Surg 1976; 3:85–98.

CHARACTERIZATION OF BOUTONNIÈRE DEFORMITY

STAGE	DESCRIPTION
I (Mild)	Slight lag (10 to 15 degrees) in PIP joint extension; DIP joint may be slightly hyperextended; MP joint is normal, minimal functional impairment
II (Moderate)	Flexion of PIP joint reaches 30 to 40 degrees; MP joint hyperextension
III (Severe)	PIP joint can no longer be extended passively

In mild cases of boutonnière deformity, the condition can be corrected passively with splinting and injections. Severe deformities represent a fixed joint and may require salvage surgery.

DIP, distal interphalangeal; MP, metacarpophalangeal; PIP, proximal interphalangeal.

From Nalebuff EA, Millender LH: Surgical treatment of the swan-neck deformity in rheumatoid arthritis. Orthop Clin North Am 1975; 6:733–752.

GARTLAND CLASSIFICATION OF DISTAL HUMERAL SUPRACONDYLAR FRACTURES

TYPE	DESCRIPTION
I	Nondisplaced fracture
II	Angulated fracture with an intact posterior cortex
III	Completely displaced

From Green NE, Swintkowski MF (eds): Skeletal Trauma in Children, 2nd ed. Philadelphia: W.B. Saunders, 1998:265.

MEYERS AND McKEEVER CLASSIFICATION OF PEDIATRIC FRACTURES OF THE ANTERIOR TIBIAL SPINE

TYPE	DESCRIPTION
I	Nondisplaced fracture
II	Fracture with elevation of the anterior portion of the anterior tibial spine, but with the fracture posteriorly reduced
III	Totally displaced fracture

From Green NE, Swintkowski MF (eds): Skeletal Trauma in Children, 2nd ed. Philadelphia: W.B. Saunders, 1998:446.

OGDEN CLASSIFICATION OF PEDIATRIC TIBIAL TUBERCLE FRACTURES

TYPE	DESCRIPTION
I	The fracture line exits through the distal portion of the ossified tibial tubercle
II	The fracture exits anteriorly, parallel with the proximal tibial physis
III	The fracture exits intraarticularly (Salter-Harris Type III)

From Green NE, Swintkowski MF (eds): Skeletal Trauma in Children, 2nd ed. Philadelphia: W.B. Saunders, 1998:448.

STEWART-MILFORD CLASSIFICATION OF HIP DISLOCATIONS

GRADE	DESCRIPTION
I	No acetabular fracture or only a minor chip
II	Posterior rim fracture, but stable after reduction
III	Posterior rim fracture with hip instability after reduction
IV	Dislocation accompanied by fracture of the femoral head and neck

From Green NE, Swintkowski MF (eds): **Skeletal Trauma in Children,** *2nd ed. Philadelphia:* **W.B. Saunders, 1998:398.**

CLASSIFICATION OF PEDIATRIC OLECRANON FRACTURES

TYPE	DESCRIPTION
I	Undisplaced, no associated injury
II	Undisplaced with fracture of proximal radius or supracondylar fracture
III	Undisplaced but with soft tissue damage (e.g., neurovascular damage)
IV	Displaced fracture

From Green NE, Swintkowski MF (eds): **Skeletal Trauma in Children,** *2nd ed. Philadelphia:* **W.B. Saunders, 1998:309.**

CLASSIFICATION OF PEDIATRIC FRACTURES OF THE MEDIAL EPICONDYLE

TYPE	DESCRIPTION
I	Undisplaced
II	Minimally displaced (<5 mm)
III	Displaced (>5 mm)
	Elbow not dislocated or reduced
	Epicondyle not in joint
	Epicondyle in joint
	Elbow dislocated

From Green NE, Swintkowski MF (eds): **Skeletal Trauma in Children,** *2nd ed. Philadelphia:* **W.B. Saunders, 1998:298.**

MILCH CLASSIFICATION OF PEDIATRIC FRACTURES OF THE LATERAL CONDYLE OF THE DISTAL HUMERUS

TYPE	DESCRIPTION
I	The fracture line is lateral to the trochlear groove, and the elbow joint does not dislocate.
II	The fracture line is at or medial to the trochlear groove, and the elbow does dislocate.

From Green NE, Swintkowski MF (eds): Skeletal Trauma in Children, 2nd ed. Philadelphia: W.B. Saunders, 1998:285.

LETTS AND ROWHANI CLASSIFICATION OF PEDIATRIC GALEAZZI FRACTURES

▷ Radius shaft fracture with dislocation of the distal radioulnar joint

TYPE		DESCRIPTION
A		Fracture of the radius at the junction of the middle and distal thirds with:
	1	Dorsal dislocation of the distal ulna
	2	Epiphyseal fracture of the distal ulna with dorsal displacement of ulnar metaphysis
B		Fracture of the distal third of the radius with:
	1	Dorsal dislocation of the distal ulna
	2	Epiphyseal fracture of the distal ulna with dorsal displacement of ulnar metaphysis
C		Greenstick fracture of the radius with dorsal bowing and:
	1	Dorsal dislocation of the distal ulna
	2	Epiphyseal fracture of the distal ulna with displacement of ulnar metaphysis
D		Fracture of distal radius with volar bowing and:
	1	Volar dislocation of distal ulna
	2	Epiphyseal fracture of the distal ulna with volar displacement of ulnar metaphysis

From Green NE, Swintkowski MF (eds): Skeletal Trauma in Children, 2nd ed. Philadelphia: W.B. Saunders, 1998:229.

DENIS' CLASSIFICATION OF SPINAL FRACTURE-DISLOCATION

TYPE	DESCRIPTION
A	Flexion-rotation injury, through either bone or disc, with three-column disruption
B	Shear injury, producing either anterior or posterior spondylolisthesis
C	Bilateral facet dislocation

From Browner BD, Jupiter JB, Levine AM, Trafton PG: Skeletal Trauma, 2nd ed. Philadelphia: W.B. Saunders, 1998:980.

DENIS' CLASSIFICATION OF VERTEBRAL BURST FRACTURES

TYPE	DESCRIPTION
A	Burst fractures involving both endplates
B	Fractures involving the superior endplate only
C	Fractures involving the inferior endplate only
D	Type A fracture with rotation
E	Fracture due to a laterally directed force that appears asymmetric on anteroposterior radiographs; one or both endplates may be involved.

From Browner BD, Jupiter JB, Levine AM, Trafton PG: Skeletal Trauma, 2nd ed. Philadelphia: W.B. Saunders, 1998:975.

DENIS' CLASSIFICATION OF COMPRESSION FRACTURES OF THE THORACIC AND LUMBAR VERTEBRAE

TYPE	DESCRIPTION
A	Fractures involving both endplates
B	Fractures involving the superior endplate only
C	Fractures involving the inferior endplate only
D	Fractures involving a buckling of the anterior cortex with both endplates intact

From Browner BD, Jupiter JB, Levine AM, Trafton PG: Skeletal Trauma, 2nd ed. Philadelphia: W.B. Saunders, 1998:968.

LEVINE AND EDWARDS CLASSIFICATION OF TRAUMATIC SPONDYLOLISTHESIS OF THE AXIS

TYPE	DESCRIPTION
I	A fracture through the neural arch with no angulation and as much as 3 mm of displacement
II	Fractures with significant angulation and displacement
IIA	Fractures with minimal displacement but severe angulation
III	Fractures with severe angulation and displacement as well as concomitant unilateral or bilateral facet dislocations at the level of C2 and C3

Type I fractures are stable, whereas the others are unstable. Type II fractures are the most common.

From Browner BD, Jupiter JB, Levine AM, Trafton PG: Skeletal Trauma, 2nd ed. Philadelphia: W.B. Saunders, 1998:879–880.

LEVINE AND EDWARDS MODIFICATION OF THE FIELDING CLASSIFICATION OF ATLANTOAXIAL ROTARY SUBLUXATION

TYPE	DESCRIPTION
I	Rotary fixation without anterior displacement at the atlas, with the atlantodental interval less than 3 mm. This is the most common type.
II	Rotary fixation with anterior displacement of the atlas of 3 to 5 mm.
III	Rotary fixation with anterior displacement greater than 5 mm of the atlas on the axis.
IV	Rotary fixation with posterior displacement of the atlas on the axis. It is seen with a deficient dens and is uncommon.
V	Frank rotary dislocation, also very uncommon.

From Browner BD, Jupiter JB, Levine AM, Trafton PG: Skeletal Trauma, 2nd ed. Philadelphia: W.B. Saunders, 1998:872.

FRANKEL CLASSIFICATION OF NEUROLOGIC DEFICIT

TYPE	DESCRIPTION
A	Absent motor and sensory function
B	Sensation present, motor function absent
C	Sensation present, motor function active but not useful (grades 2/5 to 3/5)
D	Sensation present, motor function active and useful (grade 4/5)
E	Normal motor and sensory function

This system is useful for following the progression of recovery from neural injury. Improvements of one Frankel grade are very significant.

From Browner BD, Jupiter JB, Levine AM, Trafton PG: Skeletal Trauma, 2nd ed. Philadelphia: W.B. Saunders, 1998:751.

CHRONIC REGIONAL PAIN SYNDROMES (CRPS) CLASSIFICATION

TYPE	DESCRIPTION
I	A syndrome that develops after an initiating event, is not limited to the distribution of a single peripheral nerve, and is disproportionate to the inciting event. There is continuing pain, allodynia, or hyperalgesia. In addition, there is edema, changes in skin blood flow, or abnormal sudomotor activity in the region of the pain. Also known as reflex sympathetic dystrophy (RSD).
II	A syndrome of burning pain, allodynia, and hyperpathia, usually in the hand or foot after partial injury of a nerve or one of its branches. Onset soon after injury. Usual nerves are median, sciatic, tibial, and ulnar. Also known as causalgia.

These are difficult syndromes to deal with clinically, but differentiating between the two types of CRPS may facilitate treatment.

From Browner BD, Jupiter JB, Levine AM, Trafton PG: Skeletal Trauma, 2nd ed. Philadelphia: W.B. Saunders, 1998:604–605.

CLASSIFICATION OF FRACTURES OF THE ATLAS

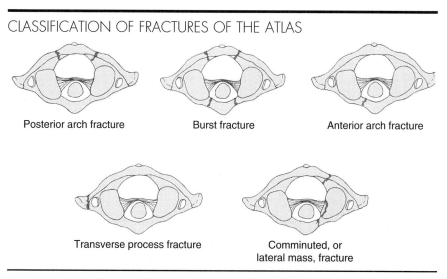

Posterior arch fracture   Burst fracture   Anterior arch fracture

Transverse process fracture   Comminuted, or lateral mass, fracture

From Browner BD, Jupiter JB, Levine AM, Trafton PG: Skeletal Trauma, 2nd ed. Philadelphia: W.B. Saunders, 1998:866.

SACRAL FRACTURE CLASSIFICATION

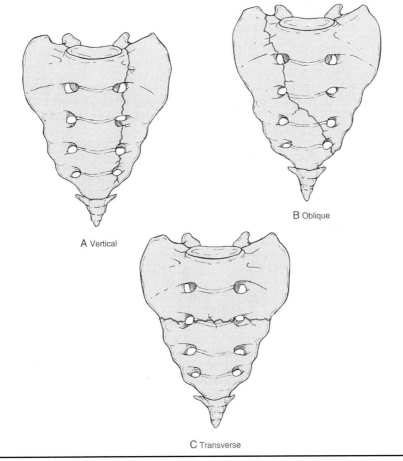

A Vertical

B Oblique

C Transverse

From Browner BD, Jupiter JB, Levine AM, Trafton PG: Skeletal Trauma, 2nd ed.
Philadelphia: W.B. Saunders, 1998:1054.

STAGES OF RHEUMATOID JOINT INVOLVEMENT

STAGE	DESCRIPTION
I	Synovitis without deformity
II	Synovitis with passively correctable deformity
III	Fixed deformity without joint changes
IV	Articular destruction

From Green DP, Hotchkiss RN, Pederson WC: Green's Operative Hand Surgery, 4th ed.
Philadelphia: Churchill Livingstone, 1999:1653.

LETOURNEL CLASSIFICATION OF ACETABULAR FRACTURES

TYPE	DESCRIPTION
A	Posterior wall fracture
B	Posterior column fracture
C	Anterior wall fracture
D	Anterior column fracture
E	Transverse fracture
F	Associated posterior column and posterior wall fractures
G	Associated transverse and posterior wall fractures
H	T-Shaped fractures
I	Associated anterior and posterior hemitransverse fractures
J	Both-column fractures

From Browner BD, Jupiter JB, Levine AM, Trafton PG: Skeletal Trauma, 2nd ed. Philadelphia: W.B. Saunders, 1998:1184–1185.

LETOURNEL CLASSIFICATION OF PELVIC FRACTURES

This is an anatomic classification scheme, and combinations will occur.

A	Iliac wing
B	Ilium with extension to the sacroiliac joint
C	Transsacral
D	Unilateral sacral fractures
E	Sacroiliac joint fracture-dislocations
F	Acetabular fractures
G	Pubic rami fractures
H	Ischial fractures
I	Pubic symphysis separation

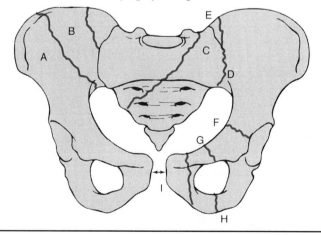

From Browner BD, Jupiter JB, Levine AM, Trafton PG: Skeletal Trauma, 2nd ed. Philadelphia: W.B. Saunders, 1998:1126.

SALTER-HARRIS CLASSIFICATION OF PHYSEAL INJURIES

TYPE	DESCRIPTION
I	Complete separation of the epiphysis and physis from the metaphysis, with fracture through the zone of hypertrophic cells
II	Similar to Type I, except that a metaphyseal fragment is present on the compression side of the fracture (Thurston-Holland sign)
III	Physeal separation with fracture through the epiphysis into the joint
IV	Fracture through the metaphysis, physis, and epiphysis into the joint
V	Compression or crushing injury to the physis
VI*	Avulsion injury to the peripheral portion of the physis, resulting in angulation due to a bony bridge of tissue

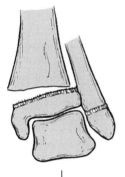

I

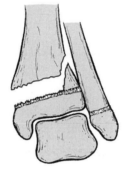

II

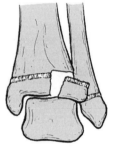

III

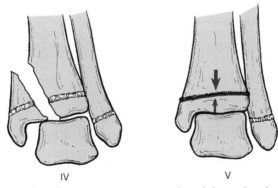

IV

V

The Salter-Harris classification system is used widely in the description of pediatric fractures. X-rays are used to determine the fracture pattern. Type II injuries are most common.

* Type VI added by Dr. Mercer Rang, Toronto, Canada.

From Green NE, Swintkowski MF (eds): Skeletal Trauma in Children, 2nd ed. Philadelphia: W.B. Saunders, 1998:22,25.

VENN-WATSON CLASSIFICATION OF POLYDACTYLY

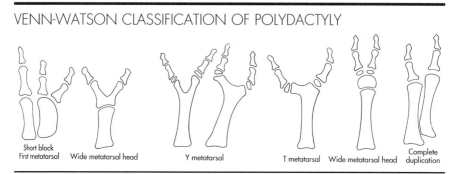

Short block
First metatarsal   Wide metatarsal head   Y metatarsal   T metatarsal   Wide metatarsal head   Complete duplication

Illustration from Canale ST (ed): Campbell's Operative Orthopedics, 9th ed. St. Louis: Mosby, 1998:927. Classification from Venn-Watson EA: Problems in polydactyly of the foot. Orthop Clin North Am 1976; 7:909.

BOYES' CLASSIFICATION OF POSTOPERATIVE HAND RECOVERY

GRADE	DESCRIPTION
1	Good. Minimal scar with mobile joints and no trophic changes.
2	Cicatrix. Heavy skin scarring due to injury or prior surgery. Deep scarring due to failed primary repair or infection.
3	Joint damage. Injury to the joint with restricted range of motion.
4	Nerve damage. Injury to the digital nerves resulting in trophic changes in the finger.
5	Multiple damage. Involvement of multiple fingers with a combination of the above problems.

From Boyes JH: Flexor tendon grafts in the fingers and thumb: An evaluation of end results. J Bone Joint Surg 1950; 32A:489–499.

CHARACTERIZATION OF SWAN-NECK DEFORMITY

TYPE	DESCRIPTION
I	PIP joints flexible in all positions
II	PIP joint flexion limited in certain positions
III	Limited PIP joint flexion in all positions
IV	Stiff PIP joints with poor radiographic appearance

The functional loss associated with swan-neck deformity is related to the loss of motion at the PIP joint.

PIP, proximal interphalangeal.

From Green DP, Hotchkiss RN, Pederson WC: Green's Operative Hand Surgery, 4th ed. Philadelphia: Churchill Livingstone, 1999:1706–1715.

ZAPICO CLASSIFICATION OF LUNATE SHAPE

TYPE	DESCRIPTION
I	Seen in ulna-minus wrists; the bone has a proximal apex or crest
II	Seen in zero variant wrists; the bone is rectangular
III	Seen in ulna-plus wrists; the bone is rectangular

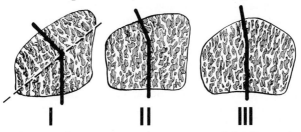

I   II   III

In Kienböck's disease, there is avascular necrosis of the lunate bone that leads to collapse of the wrist. It is thought that patients with an ulna-minus wrist (ulna proximal to the radius) are predisposed to the condition. The shape of the bone and its trabecular pattern also are thought to play a role in the development of Kienböck's disease, with Type I lunates associated with the condition.

Text from Zapico JM: Malacia del semilunar. Doctoral thesis. Universidad de Valladolid. Industrias y editorial sever cuesta, Valladolid, Spain, 1966. Illustration from Teleisnik J: The Wrist. New York: Churchill Livingstone, 1985.

WAKE FOREST CLASSIFICATION OF OCCLUSIVE/VASOSPASTIC/VASO-OCCLUSIVE DISEASE

GROUP		DESCRIPTION	ETIOLOGY
I		Raynaud's disease	Idiopathic
II		Raynaud's phenomenon	Collagen vascular disease
	A	Adequate circulation	
	B	Inadequate circulation	
III		Secondary vasospasm/occlusive disease	Vascular injury
	A	Adequate collateral circulation	Occlusion/embolus
	B	Inadequate collateral circulation	
IV		Secondary vasospasm	Nonvascular injury Nerve/bone/soft tissue damage

From Green DP, Hotchkiss RN, Pederson WC: Green's Operative Hand Surgery, 4th ed. Philadelphia: Churchill Livingstone, 1999:2278.

MALLET FINGER CLASSIFICATION

TYPE	DESCRIPTION
I	Closed or blunt trauma with loss of tendon continuity with or without a small avulsion fracture
II	Laceration at or proximal to the distal interphalangeal joint with loss of tendon continuity
III	Deep abrasion with loss of skin, subcutaneous cover, and tendon substance
IV-A	Transepiphyseal plate fracture in children
IV-B	Hyperflexion injury with fracture of the articular surface of 20% to 50%
IV-C	Hyperextension injury with fracture of the articular surface usually greater than 50% and with early or late volar subluxation of the distal phalanx

The most common type of mallet finger is Type I, and splinting of the distal interphalangeal joint in slight hyperextension may correct the deformity and obviate the need for surgery.

From Green DP, Hotchkiss RN, Pederson WC: Green's **Operative Hand Surgery, 4th ed.** *Philadelphia: Churchill Livingstone, 1999:1963.*

CHARACTERIZATION OF RHEUMATOID THUMB

TYPE	DESCRIPTION
I	Boutonnière deformity—MP joint flexion and distal joint hyperextension. This can be classified as early (passively correctable MP joint subluxation with IP joint hyperextension), moderate (fixed MP joint with passively correctable IP joint), or advanced (both MP and IP joints are fixed).
II	A combination of Type I and III deformities—MP joint flexion with IP joint hyperextension and subluxation/dislocation of the CMC joint.
III	Swan-neck deformity—MP joint hyperextension, IP joint flexion, and metacarpal adduction.
IV	Gamekeeper's deformity—radial deviation deformity of the MP joint with secondary adduction of the thumb metacarpal. There is no CMC joint disease.
V	MP joint hyperextension with secondary flexion of the IP joint as tension on the flexor tendon increases. Unlike Type III, the metacarpal is not adducted.

CMC, carpometacarpal; IP, interphalangeal; MP, metacarpophalangeal.

From Green DP, Hotchkiss RN, Pederson WC: Green's **Operative Hand Surgery, 4th ed.** *Philadelphia: Churchill Livingstone, 1999:1721–1725.*

CLASSIFICATION OF TRIGGER FINGER

GRADE	DESCRIPTION
I	Pretriggering—pain, history of catching, but not demonstrable on physical examination, tenderness over the A1 pulley
II	Active—demonstrable catching, but the patient can actively extend the digit
III	Passive—demonstrable catching requiring passive extension (Grade IIIA) or inability to actively flex (Grade IIIB)
IV	Contracture—demonstrable catching with a fixed flexion contracture of the proximal interphalangeal joint

Trigger finger is found more often in women than in men, and the most common digit is the thumb, followed by the ring, long, little, and index fingers. Secondary trigger finger is observed in patients with diabetes and rheumatoid arthritis.

From Green DP, Hotchkiss RN, Pederson WC: Green's Operative Hand Surgery, 4th ed. Philadelphia: Churchill Livingstone, 1999:2029.

WEISS-HASTINGS CLASSIFICATION OF PROXIMAL PHALANX UNICONDYLAR FRACTURES

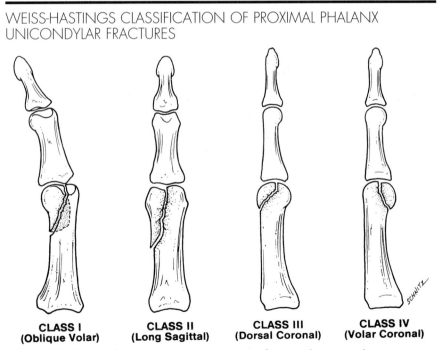

CLASS I	CLASS II	CLASS III	CLASS IV
(Oblique Volar)	(Long Sagittal)	(Dorsal Coronal)	(Volar Coronal)

Almost all of these fractures require operative fixation because they are very unstable.

From Weiss APC, Hastings H II: Distal unicondylar fractures of the proximal phalanx. J Hand Surg 1993; 18A:594–599.

EXTENSOR TENDON ZONES OF INJURY

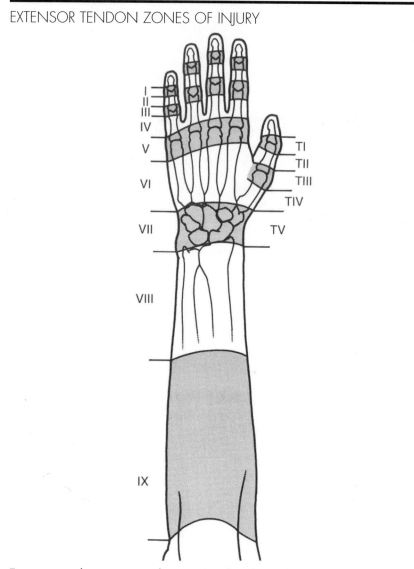

Extensor tendon injuries, when repaired early and properly, usually heal well and postoperative function is almost always good. Proximal injuries (Zones V to VIII) do better than distal injuries (Zones I to IV). Often with extensor tendon injuries, the loss of joint flexion is more severe than the loss of extension.

From Green DP, Hotchkiss RN, Pederson WC: Green's Operative Hand Surgery, 4th ed. Philadelphia: Churchill Livingstone, 1999:1956.

FERNANDEZ CLASSIFICATION OF DISTAL RADIUS FRACTURES BY MECHANISM OF INJURY

TYPE	DESCRIPTION
I	Extraarticular metaphyseal bending injuries, such as Colles' (dorsal angulation) and Smith's (volar angulation) fractures
II	Intraarticular fractures caused by shearing, such as Barton's fractures and radial styloid fractures
III	Intraarticular fractures caused by compression, such as radial pilon fractures
IV	Avulsion fractures of ligament attachments that occur with radiocarpal fracture-dislocations
V	High-velocity injuries with extensive injury

From Canale ST (ed): **Campbell's Operative Orthopedics, 9th ed. St. Louis: Mosby, 1998:2353.**

CLASSIFICATION OF KNEE JOINT INSTABILITY RESULTING FROM LIGAMENT INJURY

TYPE		DESCRIPTION
I		One-plane instability (simple or straight)
	IA	One plane medial
	IB	One plane lateral
	IC	One plane posterior
	ID	One plane anterior
II		Rotary instability
	IIA	Anteromedial
	IIB	Anterolateral
	IIB1	In flexion
	IIB2	Approaching extension
	IIC	Posterolateral
	IID	Posteromedial
III		Combined instability
	IIIA	Anterolateral-anteromedial rotary
	IIIB	Anterolateral-posterolateral rotary
	IIIC	Anteromedial-posteromedial rotary

From Canale ST (ed): **Campbell's Operative Orthopedics, 9th ed. St. Louis: Mosby, 1998:1168.**

HOHL AND MOORE CLASSIFICATION OF TIBIAL PLATEAU FRACTURES

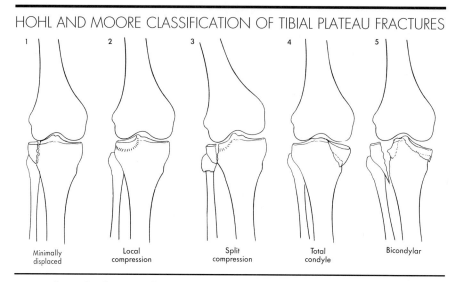

| Minimally displaced | Local compression | Split compression | Total condyle | Bicondylar |

Illustration from Canale ST (ed): Campbell's Operative Orthopedics, 9th ed. St. Louis: Mosby, 1998:2095. Classification scheme from Hohl M, Moore TM: Articular fractures of the proximal tibia. In Evarts CM (ed): Surgery of the Musculoskeletal System, 2nd ed. New York: Churchill Livingstone, 1990.

CLASSIFICATION OF CAPITELLAR FRACTURES

TYPE	DESCRIPTION
1	A large fragment of bone and articular cartilage is present
2	A small shell of bone and articular cartilage is present
3	The fracture is comminuted

From Canale ST (ed): Campbell's Operative Orthopedics, 9th ed. St. Louis: Mosby, 1998:2320.

RUEDI AND ALLGOWER CLASSIFICATION OF DISTAL TIBIAL ARTICULAR FRACTURES

TYPE	DESCRIPTION
I	Nondisplaced cleavage fractures that involve the joint surface
II	Cleave-type fracture lines with displacement of the articular surface but minimal comminution
III	Fractures associated with metaphyseal and articular comminution

From Canale ST (ed): Campbell's Operative Orthopedics, 9th ed. St. Louis: Mosby, 1998:2057.

MÜLLER CLASSIFICATION OF DISTAL FEMUR FRACTURES

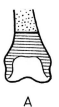

A

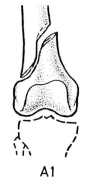

A1

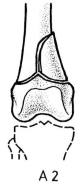

A 2

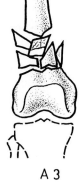

A 3

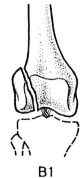

B

B1

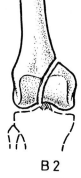

B 2

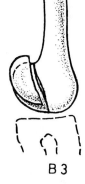

B 3

C

C1

C 2

C 3

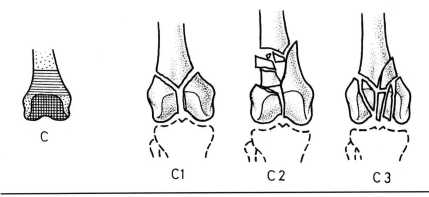

Illustration from Canale ST (ed): Campbell's Operative Orthopedics, 9th ed. St. Louis: Mosby, 1998:2121. Scheme from Müller ME, Nazarian S, Koch P, Schatzker J: The Comprehensive Classification of Fractures of Long Bones. Berlin: Springer-Verlag, 1990.

BADO CLASSIFICATION OF MONTEGGIA FRACTURES
▷ Ulnar fracture with dislocation of the proximal end of the radius with or without radial fractures

TYPE	DESCRIPTION
1	Fracture of the middle or proximal third of the ulna with anterior dislocation of the radial head and characteristic apex angulation of the ulna
2	Fracture of the middle or proximal third of the ulna (the apex is usually posteriorly angulated) with posterior dislocation of the radial head and often a fracture of the radial head
3	Fracture of the ulna just distal to the coronoid process with lateral dislocation of the radial head
4	Fracture of the proximal or middle third of the ulna, anterior dislocation of the radial head, and fracture of the proximal third of the radius below the bicipital tuberosity

Type 1 fractures are the most common by far.

From Canale ST (ed): Campbell's Operative Orthopedics, **9th ed. St. Louis: Mosby, 1998:2332.**

TRIANGULAR FIBROCARTILAGE COMPLEX (TFCC) ABNORMALITIES

CLASS I—TRAUMATIC
A. Central perforation
B. Medial avulsion (ulnar attachment) with or without distal ulnar fracture
C. Distal avulsion (carpal attachment)
D. Lateral avulsion (radial attachment) with or without sigmoid notch fracture

CLASS II—DEGENERATIVE
Stage 1 TFCC wear
Stage 2 TFCC wear + lunate and/or ulnar chondromalacia
Stage 3 TFCC perforation + lunate and/or ulnar chondromalacia
Stage 4 TFCC perforation + lunate and/or ulnar chondromalacia + L-T ligament perforation
Stage 5 TFCC perforation + lunate and/or ulnar chondromalacia + L-T ligament perforation + ulnocarpal arthritis

From Palmer AK: Triangular fibrocartilage complex lesions: A classification. J Hand Surg 1989; 14A:594–606.

FRYKMAN CLASSIFICATION OF DISTAL RADIUS FRACTURES

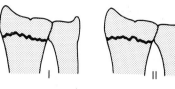

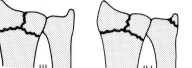

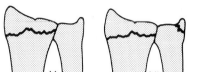

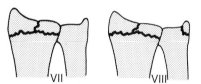

The higher the grade, the more complex the fracture and the worse the prognosis becomes.

From Green DP, Hotchkiss RN, Pederson WC: Green's Operative Hand Surgery, 4th ed. Philadelphia: Churchill Livingstone, 1999:935.

RUSSE CLASSIFICATION OF SCAPHOID FRACTURES

Horizontal oblique
Transverse
Vertical oblique

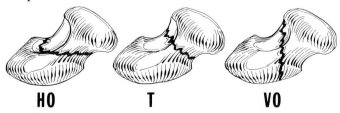

HO   **T**   **VO**

Horizontal oblique and transverse fractures tend to be stable and usually heal without incident. Vertical oblique fractures are much more unstable.

From Teleisnik J: The Wrist. New York: Churchill Livingstone, 1985.

CLASSIFICATION OF ROTARY SUBLUXATION OF THE SCAPHOID (RSS)

TYPE	DESCRIPTION
I	Predynamic RSS—signs and symptoms of scaphoid instability exist without radiographic abnormalities
II	Dynamic RSS—signs and symptoms of RSS with positive findings on stress radiographic views (clenched fist, radial or ulnar deviation)
III	Static RSS—signs and symptoms of RSS and positive findings on routine posteroanterior and lateral radiographs
IV	Degenerative RSS—severe symptoms of RSS with a longer duration and usually in an older patient
V	Secondary RSS—involvement of the scaphoid secondary to other carpal lesions

*From Green DP, Hotchkiss RN, Pederson WC: Green's **Operative Hand Surgery, 4th ed.** Philadelphia: Churchill Livingstone, 1999:110.*

FLEXOR TENDON ZONES OF INJURY

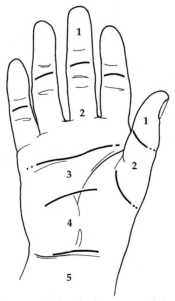

Zone 2 is considered "no man's land" because of the difficulty in restoring normal tendon gliding to injuries in this zone.

*From Marks MW, Marks C (eds): **Fundamentals of Plastic Surgery.** Philadelphia: W.B. Saunders, 1997:356.*

OGDEN CLASSIFICATION OF PHYSEAL INJURIES COMPARED WITH POLAND AND SALTER-HARRIS CLASSIFICATIONS

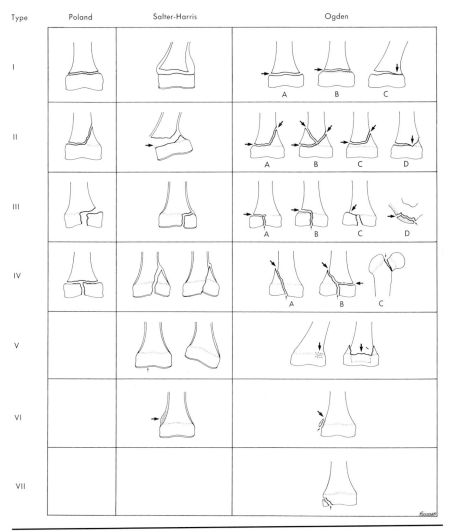

| Type | Poland | Salter-Harris | Ogden |

From Crenshaw (ed): Campbell's Operative Orthopedics, 7th ed. St. Louis: Mosby, 1987:1835.

COMPREHENSIVE CLASSIFICATION OF PELVIC RING DISRUPTIONS

TYPE A—STABLE, POSTERIOR ARCH INTACT

A1   Posterior arch intact, fracture of innominate bone (avulsion)
     A1.1   Iliac spine
     A1.2   Iliac crest
     A1.3   Ischial tuberosity

A2   Posterior arch intact, fracture of innominate bone (direct blow)
     A2.1   Iliac wing fractures
     A2.2   Unilateral fracture of anterior arch
     A2.3   Bifocal fracture of anterior arch

A3   Posterior arch intact, transverse fracture of sacrum caudal to S2
     A3.1   Sacrococcygeal dislocation
     A3.2   Sacrum undisplaced
     A3.3   Sacrum displaced

TYPE B—INCOMPLETE DISRUPTION OF POSTERIOR ARCH, PARTIALLY STABLE, ROTATION

B1   External rotation instability, open-book injury, unilateral
     B1.1   Sacroiliac joint, anterior disruption
     B1.2   Sacral fracture

B2   Incomplete disruption of posterior arch, unilateral, internal rotation
     B2.1   Anterior compression fracture, sacrum
     B2.2   Partial sacroiliac joint fracture, subluxation
     B2.3   Incomplete posterior iliac fracture

B3   Incomplete disruption of posterior arch, bilateral
     B3.1   Bilateral open-book
     B3.2   Open-book, lateral compression
     B3.3   Bilateral lateral compression

TYPE C—COMPLETE DISRUPTION OF POSTERIOR ARCH, UNSTABLE

C1   Complete disruption of posterior arch, unilateral
     C1.1   Fracture through ilium
     C1.2   Sacroiliac dislocation and/or fracture dislocation
     C1.3   Sacral fracture

C2   Bilateral injury, one side rotationally unstable, one side vertically unstable

C3   Bilateral injury, both sides completely unstable

From Browner BD, Jupiter JB, Levine AM, Trafton PG: Skeletal Trauma, 2nd ed. Philadelphia: W.B. Saunders, 1998:1129.

LEDDY AND PACKER CLASSIFICATION OF PROFUNDUS TENDON AVULSION INJURIES

TYPE	DESCRIPTION
I	The tendon retracts into the palm
II	The tendon retracts to the level of the proximal interphalangeal joint—a small fragment may be seen on lateral x-ray
III	A large bony fragment is avulsed that is connected to the profundus stump and retracts to the level of the A4 pulley

TYPE I — PROFUNDUS IN PALM

TYPE II — SMALL FRAGMENT AT A3 PULLEY

TYPE III — LARGE DISTAL FRAGMENT

A Type II injury may convert to a Type I if not immediately treated. Old, untreated avulsions usually are not candidates for reinsertion because the muscle-tendon unit is chronically shortened.

From Leddy JR, Packer JW: Avulsion of the profundus tendon insertion in athletes. J Hand Surg (Am) 1977; 2:66–69.

AMERICAN SPINAL INJURY ASSOCIATION (ASIA) SCALE OF SPINAL CORD INJURY

Five motor groups in the upper extremity (biceps, wrist extensors, triceps, flexor profundus and intrinsics) and five motor groups in the lower extremity (iliopsoas, quadriceps, tibialis anterior, extensor hallucis longus and gastrocnemius) are tested bilaterally.

GRADE	FUNCTION
0	Absent function
1	Trace
2	Active without gravity
3	Active against gravity
4	Active against resistance
5	Normal motor function

Sum of all four quadrants is 0 (tetraplegia) to 100 (normal)

From Browner BD, Jupiter JB, Levine AM, Trafton PG: **Skeletal Trauma, 2nd ed.** *Philadelphia: W.B. Saunders, 1998:841.*

CLINICAL SCALE OF MOTOR CONTROL

GRADE	MOTOR CONTROL	DESCRIPTION
1	Flaccid	Hypotonic, no active motion
2	Rigid	Hypertonic, no active motion
3	Reflexive mass pattern	Mass flexion or extension in response to stimulation
4	Volitional mass pattern	Patient-initiated mass flexion or extension movement
5	Selective with pattern overlay	Slow volitional movement of specific joints; physiologic stress results in mass action
6	Selective	Volitional control of individual joints

From Keenan MA: Stroke. In Kasser JR (ed): **Orthopaedic Knowledge Update 5.** *Rosemont, IL: American Academy of Orthopaedic Surgeons, 1996:689–693.*

SUD CLASSIFICATION OF METAPHYSEAL FRACTURES

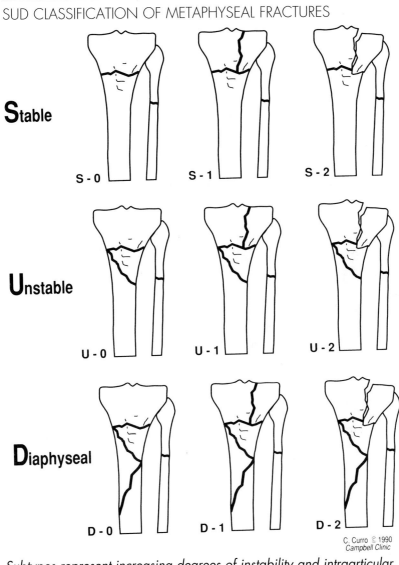

Subtypes represent increasing degrees of instability and intraarticular extension.

From Gustilo RB, Kyle RF, Templeman DC: **Fractures and Dislocations.** *St. Louis: Mosby,* 1993.

ORTHOPEDIC TRAUMA ASSOCIATION CLASSIFICATION OF LONG BONE FRACTURES

Linear

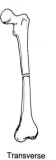 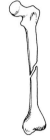 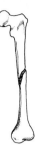

Transverse   Oblique   Spiral

Comminuted

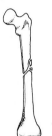 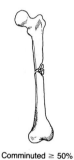

Comminuted ≤ 50%   Comminuted ≥ 50%   Butterfly < 50%   Butterfly ≥ 50%

Segmental

Two Level   Three Levels or More   Longitudinal Split   Comminuted

Bone loss

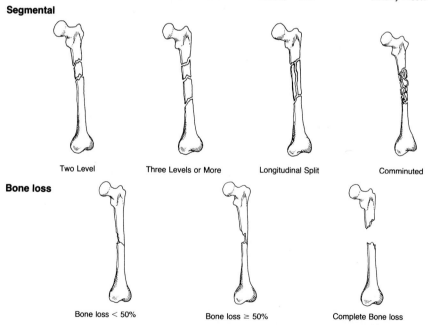

Bone loss < 50%   Bone loss ≥ 50%   Complete Bone loss

From Gustilo RB: **The Fracture Classification Manual.** *St. Louis: Mosby, 1991.*

CLASSIFICATION OF CLOSED FRACTURES WITH SOFT TISSUE INJURIES

TYPE	DESCRIPTION
0	Minimal soft tissue damage. Indirect violence. Simple fracture patterns. Example: torsion fracture of the tibia in skiers.
I	Superficial abrasion or contusion caused by pressure from within. Mild to moderately severe fracture configuration. Example: pronation fracture-dislocation of the ankle joint with soft tissue lesion over the medial malleolus.
II	Deep, contaminated abrasion associated with localized skin or muscle contusion. Impending compartment syndrome. Severe fracture configuration. Example: segmental "bumper" fracture of the tibia.
III	Extensive skin contusion or crush. Underlying muscle damage may be severe. Subcutaneous avulsion. Decompensated compartment syndrome. Associated major vascular injury. Severe or comminuted fracture configuration.

From Tscherne H, Oestern H-J: Die Klassifizierung des Weichteilschadens bei offenen und geschlossenen Frakturen. Unfallheikunde 1982; 85:111–115.

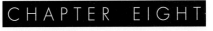

Head and Neck Surgery

GRADING OF TONSILLAR ENLARGEMENT

GRADE	DESCRIPTION
1	Tonsil tissue is very small and insignificant
2	Tonsil tissue is normal and nonobstructive
3	Tonsils are large and appear to crowd the oropharynx
4	Tonsils completely fill the oropharynx with flat medial surfaces opposing each other

BRODSKY SCHEME OF GRADING TONSILLAR ENLARGEMENT

GRADE	DESCRIPTION
0	Tonsils do not encroach the airway
+1	Tonsils occlude <25% of the airway
+2	Tonsils are readily apparent and obstructing 25% to 50% of the airway
+3	Tonsils obstruct 50% to 75% of the airway
+4	Tonsils are massive and obstruct >75% of the airway

From Meyerhoff WL, Rice DH (eds): Otolaryngology—Head and Neck Surgery. Philadelphia: W.B. Saunders, 1992:656.

GRADING OF LARYNGEAL STENOSIS

GRADE	LARYNGEAL LUMEN OBSTRUCTION
I	<50%
II	51% to 70%
III	71% to 99%
IV	Complete obstruction

Endoscopy is used to measure the laryngeal diameter and provide information about vocal cord function.

From Bailey BJ, Calhoun KH, Coffey AR, Neely JG (eds): Head and Neck Surgery— Otolaryngology. Philadelphia: Lippincott-Raven, 1998:1117.

HANNA CLASSIFICATION OF HEAD AND NECK DEFECTS

CLASS	DESCRIPTION
A	Defects requiring mandatory coverage (brain, great vessels, etc.)
B	Defects yielding major functional deficits (oral cavity, lips, facial nerve, etc.)
C	Defects yielding aesthetic deficits (nose, eyes, etc.)

From Hanna DC: Present and future trends in reconstructive surgery for head and neck cancer patients. Laryngoscope 1978; 88(Suppl 8):96–100.

CLASSIFICATION OF TYMPANOMETRIC PATTERNS

TYPE	TYMPANIC MEMBRANE	CORRELATION
A	Normal compliance	Normal
A_s	Stiff	Otosclerosis
A_d	Hypermobile	Discontinuous ear bones
C	Negative middle ear pressure	Eustachian tube malfunction Otitis media recovery
B	Retracted, immobile, noncompliant membrane	Middle ear effusion Ear wax occlusion Membrane perforation

Data from Koufman JA: Core Otolaryngology. Philadelphia: Lippincott-Raven, 1990:47–49.

CLASSIFICATION OF CLEFT LARYNX

TYPE	DESCRIPTION
I	A supraglottic interarytenoid cleft above the level of the vocal cords
II	A partial cricoid cleft extending below the level of the vocal cords and partially through the posterior lamina of the cricoid cartilage
III	A total cricoid cleft with or without further extension into the cervical tracheoesophageal wall
IV	A laryngotracheoesophageal cleft

From Benjamin B, Inglis A: Minor congenital laryngeal clefts: Diagnosis and classification. Ann Otol Rhinol Laryngol 1989; 98:419.

STAGING OF ESOPHAGEAL BURNS

DEGREE	DESCRIPTION
1st	Mucosal erythema
2nd	Mucosal erythema
	Noncircumferential exudates
3rd	Mucosal erythema
	Circumferential exudate
4th	Mucosal erythema
	Circumferential exudate
	Esophageal wall perforation

Additional information gained at the time of endoscopy is the length of the burn and the specific site. All first-degree burns and some second-degree burns will heal without stricture.

From Estrera A, Taylor W, Mills LJ, Platt MR, et al.: Corrosive burns of the esophagus and stomach: A recommendation for an aggressive surgical approach. Ann Thorac Surg 1986; 41:276, with permission from Elsevier Science.

CLASSIFICATION OF SLEEP APNEA

GRADE	RDI	Sao_2 (%)
Mild	5–20	>85
Moderate	21–40	65–84
Severe	>40	<65

The RDI (respiratory disturbance index) is the mean number of apneas and hypopneas per hour. Each sleep center may define a hypopneic event in a different manner.

From the American Sleep Disorders Association: Sleep Apnea Committee. Sleep Apnea: Physiology and Diagnosis Slide Series, Rochester, MN, 1991.

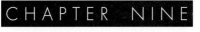

Transplant Surgery

UNITED NETWORK FOR ORGAN SHARING (UNOS) MEDICAL
URGENCY STATUS CODES FOR ADULT HEART
TRANSPLANT CANDIDATES

STATUS CODE	DESCRIPTION

1A	A patient is admitted to a transplant center hospital and has at least one of the following devices or therapies in place:
	a. Mechanical circulatory support for acute hemodynamic decompensation that includes at least one of the following:
	   i. left and/or right ventricular assist device implanted for 30 days or less
	   ii. total artificial heart
	   iii. intraaortic balloon pump
	   iv. extracorporeal membrane oxygenator
	b. Mechanical circulatory support for more than 30 days with objective medical evidence of significant device-related complication
	c. Mechanical ventilation
	d. Continuous infusion of a single high-dose intravenous inotrope, or multiple intravenous inotropes, in addition to continuous hemodynamic monitoring of left ventricular filling pressures. (Qualification for status 1A under this criterion is valid for 7 days with a 7-day renewal for each occurrence of a status 1A listing for the same patient.)
	e. A patient who does not meet the criteria specified in a, b, c, or d may be listed as status 1A if the patient is admitted to the listing transplant center hospital and has a life expectancy without a heart transplant of less than 7 days. Qualification for status 1A under this criterion is valid for 7 days and must be recertified by an attending physician every 7 days to continue the status 1A listing.

Table continued on following page

UNITED NETWORK FOR ORGAN SHARING (UNOS) MEDICAL URGENCY STATUS CODES FOR ADULT HEART TRANSPLANT CANDIDATES *Continued*

STATUS CODE	DESCRIPTION
1B	A patient listed as status 1B has at least one of the following devices or therapies in place: aa. Left and/or right ventricular assist device implanted for more than 30 days bb. Continuous infusion of intravenous inotropes
2	A patient who does not meet the criteria for status 1A or 1B
7	A patient listed as status 7 is considered temporarily unsuitable to receive a thoracic organ transplant.

From the United Network for Organ Sharing, Richmond, Virginia.

CARDIAC ALLOGRAFT BIOPSY GRADING
CELLULAR REJECTION

GRADE	DESCRIPTION	NOMENCLATURE
0	No rejection	No rejection
1A	Focal (perivascular or interstitial) cellular infiltrate without myocyte necrosis	Mild rejection
1B	Diffuse, sparse cellular infiltrate without myocyte necrosis	Mild rejection
2	Single focus with an aggressive cellular infiltrate and/or focal myocyte necrosis	"Focal" moderate rejection
3A	Multifocal aggressive infiltrates and/or myocyte necrosis	"Low" moderate rejection
3B	Diffuse cellular inflammatory process with myocyte necrosis	"Borderline" severe rejection
4	Diffuse, aggressive cellular infiltrate ± edema, ± hemorrhage, ± vasculitis with marked myocyte necrosis	Severe acute rejection

This grading system is used by the International Society for Heart/Lung Transplantation (ISHLT) to assess cardiac rejection.

From Olsen S, Wagoner L, Hammond E, et al.: Vascular rejection in heart transplantation: Clinical correlation, treatment options, and future considerations. J Heart Lung Transplant 1993; 12:S135–S142, with permission from Elsevier Science.

UNITED NETWORK FOR ORGAN SHARING (UNOS) MEDICAL URGENCY STATUS CODES FOR ADULT LIVER TRANSPLANT CANDIDATES

STATUS CODE	DESCRIPTION
7	A patient listed as status 7 is temporarily inactive; however, the patient continues to accrue waiting time up to a maximum of 30 days.
3	A patient listed as status 3 requires continuous medical care and has a Child-Turcotte-Pugh (CTP) score greater than or equal to 7. These patients may be followed at home or near the transplant center. Short hospitalizations for intercurrent problems do not change status.
2B	A patient listed as 2B has a CTP score greater than or equal to 10, or a CTP score greater than or equal to 7 and meets at least one of the following criteria: i. Documented unresponsive active variceal hemorrhage ii. Hepatorenal syndrome iii. Spontaneous bacterial peritonitis iv. Refractory ascites/hepato-hydrothorax
2A	Status 2A provides a transition for currently listed adult patients with chronic liver disease who may have qualified for status 1 as this category was defined prior to July 4, 1997. A patient listed as status 2A is in the hospital's critical care unit due to chronic liver failure with a life expectancy without liver transplant of less than 7 days, and has a long-term prognosis with a successful liver transplant equivalent to that of a patient with fulminant liver failure. The patient also has a CTP score greater than or equal to 10 and meets one of the following medical criteria: i. Documented unresponsive active variceal hemorrhage ii. Hepatorenal syndrome iii. Refractory ascites/hepato-hydrothorax iv. Stage III or IV encephalopathy unresponsive to medical therapy A patient should not be listed as status 2A if the patient meets at least one of the following medical criteria: i. Extrahepatic sepsis unresponsive to antimicrobial therapy ii. Requirement for high-dose or two or more pressors to maintain adequate blood pressure iii. Severe irreversible multi-organ system failure

Table continued on following page

UNITED NETWORK FOR ORGAN SHARING (UNOS) MEDICAL URGENCY STATUS CODES FOR ADULT LIVER TRANSPLANT CANDIDATES Continued

STATUS CODE	DESCRIPTION
1	A patient older than or equal to 18 years of age listed as status 1 has fulminant liver failure with a life expectancy without liver transplant of less than 7 days. Fulminant liver failure is defined as: i. The onset of hepatic encephalopathy within 8 weeks of the first symptom of liver disease. The absence of preexisting liver disease is critical to the diagnosis ii. Primary nonfunction of a transplanted liver within 7 days of implantation iii. Hepatic artery thrombosis in a transplanted liver within 7 days of implantation iv. Acute decompensated Wilson's disease

From the United Network for Organ Sharing, Richmond, Virginia.

CHILD-TURCOTTE-PUGH (CTP) SCORE OF LIVER FUNCTION

	1 POINT	2 POINTS	3 POINTS
Albumin (g/dL)	>3.5	2.8–3.5	<2.8
Bilirubin (mg/dL)	<2.0	2–3	>3
Prothrombin time (secs. prolonged)	<4	4–6	>6
or international normalized ratio (INR)	<1.7	1.7–2.3	>2.3
Ascites	Absent	Slight	Moderate
Encephalopathy (grade)	0	1–2	3–4
For primary biliary cirrhosis, primary sclerosing cholangitis, or other cholestatic liver disease, substitute *these values for bilirubin*	*<4*	*4–10*	*>10*

SCORE: 5–6 points Child's A
         7–9 points Child's B
         10–15 points Child's C

The CTP scoring system for liver function is considered to be a more accurate method of assigning a Child's rating than previous versions, in which a point value was not assigned. Class A patients are not candidates for liver transplantation, whereas some Class B and most Class C are candidates.

From the United Network for Organ Sharing, Richmond, Virginia.

STAGING OF HEPATIC ENCEPHALOPATHY

STAGE	MENTAL STATUS	NEUROMUSCULAR	ELECTROENCEPHALOGRAM
I	Mild confusion	Normal	Normal
II	Drowsy but speaking Incontinence Inappropriate	Asterixis Brisk reflexes Increased tone	Generalized slowing
III	Sleeping but arousable Incoherent Confused	Upgoing plantar Clonus Localized or flexion response to pain	Generalized slowing
IV	No response	Sustained clonus Extensor response to pain	Generalized slowing

Data from Fraser CL, Arieff AI: Hepatic encephalopathy. N Engl J Med 1985; 313:865–873.

BANFF CLASSIFICATION OF ACUTE RENAL ALLOGRAFT REJECTION

GRADE	BIOPSY FINDING
Normal	Normal or with minor interstitial lymphoplasmacytic infiltration
Borderline	Minor interstitial lymphoplasmacytic infiltration with occasional penetration of tubular epithelium
I	Widespread focal interstitial lymphoplasmacytic infiltration with mild tubulitis; normal glomeruli and arterial vessels
II	Extensive interstitial lymphoplasmacytic infiltration with definite tubulitis and intimal cell prominence with subintimal vacuolation in arterial vessels
III	Extensive interstitial lymphoplasmacytic infiltration with tubulitis and lymphoplasmacytic infiltration of arterial walls, sometimes accompanied by fibrinoid change or medial smooth muscle necrosis

From Solez K: International standardization of nomenclature for the histological diagnosis of renal allograft rejection: The Banff working classification of kidney transplant pathology. Kidney Int 1993; 44:411–422, reprinted by permission of Blackwell Science, Inc.

BANFF CLASSIFICATION OF CHRONIC RENAL ALLOGRAFT REJECTION

GRADE	BIOPSY FINDING
I (mild)	Mild interstitial fibrosis and tubular atrophy without (a) or with (b) specific vascular changes suggesting chronic rejection
II (moderate)	Moderate interstitial fibrosis and tubular atrophy without (a) or with (b) specific vascular changes suggesting chronic rejection
III (severe)	Severe interstitial fibrosis and tubular atrophy without (a) or with (b) specific vascular changes suggesting chronic rejection

From Solez K, Benediktsson H, Cavallo T, et al.: Report of the third Banff conference on allograft pathology (July 20–24, 1995) on classification and lesion scoring in renal allograft pathology. Transplant Proc 1996; 28:441–444, with permission from Elsevier Science.

CLASSIFICATION OF LUNG TRANSPLANT REJECTION

A. Acute rejection: perivascular inflammation
  Grade 0—none
  Grade 1—minimal: infrequent perivascular infiltrates
  Grade 2—mild: frequent perivascular infiltrates
  Grade 3—moderate: dense perivascular infiltrates extending into alveolar space
  Grade 4—severe: diffuse perivascular, interstitial, and alveolar infiltrates; pneumocyte damage, and parenchymal necrosis, infarction, or necrotizing vasculitis
With or without:
B. Airway inflammation: lymphocytic bronchitis/bronchiolitis—documented with acute rejection
  Grade 0—none
  Grade 1—minimal
  Grade 2—mild
  Grade 3—moderate
  Grade 4—severe
C. Chronic airway rejection: bronchiolitis obliterans, active or inactive
D. Chronic vascular rejection: accelerated graft vascular sclerosis
The key factor in acute rejection is the degree of perivascular lymphocytic infiltration. Chronic rejection is manifested as bronchiolitis obliterans and vascular sclerosis.

From Hopkinson DN, Bhabra MS, Hooper TL: Pulmonary graft preservation: A worldwide survey of current clinical practice. J Heart Lung Transplant 1998; 17:525–531, with permission from Elsevier Science.

STAGING OF BRONCHIOLITIS OBLITERANS

STAGE	SEVERITY	FEV_1 (% of baseline)
0	No symptoms	>80%
1	Mild	66%–80%
2	Moderate	51%–65%
3	Severe	<50%

Staging is subclassified as "a" (histologic evidence of bronchiolitis obliterans) or as "b" (no histologic evidence).

FEV_1, forced expiratory volume in 1 second.

From Theodore J, Starnes VA, Lewiston NJ: Obliterative bronchiolitis. Clin Chest Med 1990; 11:309–321.

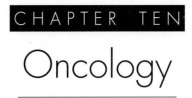

CHAPTER TEN

Oncology

CANCER STAGING

The following cancer staging schemes were developed by the American Joint Committee on Cancer (AJCC). All are based on a presumption that, in general, a cancer begins as a distinct entity, then spreads to lymph nodes, and then finally spreads to distant sites. The TNM (tumor, node, metastasis) system attempts to standardize the descriptions of all of the common cancers. Stages are basically a way of grouping the TNM combinations into "early" and "late" presentations.

The prefix c before TNM refers to the clinical stage; p before TNM refers to the pathologic stage, which includes the clinical information and information obtained from surgery and subsequent pathologic examination. The prefix r refers to retreatment and implies updated staging after a disease-free interval. Finally, an a prefix refers to classification made during an autopsy.

The pathologic stage does not replace the clinical stage; rather, the two are both left in the medical record and aid in the selection of treatment. When in doubt about the correct T, N, or M classification, use the less advanced one.

Every cancer patient should have his or her disease accurately classified and staged, and this information should be recorded in the medical record on a cancer staging form, available from the AJCC.

AMPULLA OF VATER CANCER CLASSIFICATIONS

PRIMARY TUMOR (T)

TX	Primary tumor cannot be assessed
T0	No evidence of primary tumor
Tis	Carcinoma in situ
T1	Tumor limited to the ampulla of Vater or sphincter of Oddi
T2	Tumor invades duodenal wall
T3	Tumor invades 2 cm or less into the pancreas
T4	Tumor invades more than 2 cm into pancreas and/or into other adjacent organs

REGIONAL LYMPH NODES (N)

NX	Regional lymph nodes cannot be assessed
N0	No regional lymph node metastasis
N1	Regional lymph node metastasis

DISTANT METASTASIS (M)

MX	Distant metastasis cannot be assessed
M0	No distant metastasis
M1	Distant metastasis

Stage Grouping

Stage 0	Tis	N0	M0
Stage I	T1	N0	M0
Stage II	T2	N0	M0
	T3	N0	M0
Stage III	T1	N1	M0
	T2	N1	M0
	T3	N1	M0
Stage IV	T4	Any N	M0
	Any T	Any N	M1

From AJCC Cancer Staging Handbook. Philadelphia: Lippincott-Raven, 1998:108–109.

ANAL CANAL CANCER CLASSIFICATIONS

PRIMARY TUMOR (T)

TX	Primary tumor cannot be assessed
T0	No evidence of primary tumor
Tis	Carcinoma in situ
T1	Tumor 2 cm or less in greatest dimension
T2	Tumor more than 2 cm but not more than 5 cm in greatest dimension
T3	Tumor more than 5 cm in greatest dimension
T4	Tumor of any size invades adjacent organ(s); e.g., vagina, urethra, bladder (involvement of the sphincter muscle[s] alone is not classified as T4)

REGIONAL LYMPH NODES (N)

NX	Regional lymph nodes cannot be assessed
N0	No regional lymph node metastasis
N1	Metastasis in perirectal lymph node(s)
N2	Metastasis in unilateral internal iliac and/or inguinal lymph node(s)
N3	Metastasis in perirectal and inguinal lymph nodes and/or bilateral internal iliac and/or inguinal lymph nodes

DISTANT METASTASIS (M)

MX	Distant metastasis cannot be assessed
M0	No distant metastasis
M1	Distant metastasis

Stage Grouping

Stage 0	Tis	N0	M0
Stage I	T1	N0	M0
Stage II	T2	N0	M0
	T3	N0	M0
Stage IIIA	T1	N1	M0
	T2	N1	M0
	T3	N1	M0
	T4	N0	M0
Stage IIIB	T4	N1	M0
	Any T	N2	M0
	Any T	N3	M0
Stage IV	Any T	Any N	M1

From **AJCC Cancer Staging Handbook.** *Philadelphia: Lippincott-Raven, 1998:90–91.*

BONE CANCER CLASSIFICATION

PRIMARY TUMOR (T)

TX	Primary tumor cannot be assessed
T0	No evidence of primary tumor
T1	Tumor confined within the cortex
T2	Tumor invades beyond the cortex

REGIONAL LYMPH NODES (N)

NX	Regional lymph nodes cannot be assessed
N0	No regional lymph node metastasis
N1	Regional lymph node metastasis

DISTANT METASTASIS (M)

MX	Distant metastasis cannot be assessed
M0	No distant metastasis
M1	Distant metastasis

HISTOPATHOLOGIC GRADE (G)

GX	Grade cannot be assessed
G1	Well differentiated—low grade
G2	Moderately differentiated—low grade
G3	Poorly differentiated—high grade
G4	Undifferentiated—high grade

Note: Ewing's sarcoma is classified as G4.

Stage Grouping

Stage IA	G1,2	T1	N0	M0
Stage IB	G1,2	T2	N0	M0
Stage IIA	G3,4	T1	N0	M0
Stage IIB	G3,4	T2	N0	M0
Stage III	Not defined			
Stage IVA	Any G	Any T	N1	M0
Stage IVB	Any G	Any T	Any N	M1

From **AJCC Cancer Staging Handbook.** *Philadelphia: Lippincott-Raven, 1998:136–137.*

BREAST CANCER CLASSIFICATION

PRIMARY TUMOR (T)

TX   Primary tumor cannot be assessed

T0   No evidence of primary tumor

Tis Carcinoma in situ: intraductal carcinoma, lobular carcinoma in situ, or Paget's disease of the nipple with no tumor

T1   Tumor 2 cm or less in greatest dimension

   T1mic Microinvasion 0.1 cm or less in greatest dimension

   T1a   Tumor more than 0.1 cm but not more than 0.5 cm in greatest dimension

   T1b   Tumor more than 0.5 cm but not more than 1 cm in greatest dimension

   T1c   Tumor more than 1 cm but not more than 2 cm in greatest dimension

T2   Tumor more than 2 cm but not more than 5 cm in greatest dimension

T3   Tumor more than 5 cm in greatest dimension

T4   Tumor of any size with direct extension to (a) chest wall or (b) skin, only as described below

   T4a   Extension to chest wall

   T4b   Edema (including peau d'orange) or ulceration of the skin of the breast or satellite skin nodules confined to the same breast

   T4c   Both (T4a and T4b)

   T4d   Inflammatory carcinoma

REGIONAL LYMPH NODES (N)

NX   Regional lymph nodes cannot be assessed (e.g., previously removed)

N0   No regional lymph node metastasis

N1   Metastasis to movable ipsilateral axillary lymph node(s)

N2   Metastasis to ipsilateral axillary lymph node(s) fixed to one another or to other structures

N3   Metastasis to ipsilateral internal mammary lymph node(s)

PATHOLOGIC CLASSIFICATION (pN)

pNX Regional lymph nodes cannot be assessed (e.g., previously removed, or not removed for pathologic study)

pN0 No regional lymph node metastasis

pN1 Metastasis to movable ipsilateral axillary lymph node(s)

   pN1a   Only micrometastasis (none larger than 0.2 cm)

   pN1b   Metastasis to lymph node(s), any larger than 0.2 cm

      pN1bi   Metastasis in one to three lymph nodes, any more than 0.2 cm and all less than 2 cm in greatest dimension

      pN1bii Metastasis to four or more lymph nodes, any more than 0.2 cm and all less than 2 cm in greatest dimension

Table continued on following page

BREAST CANCER CLASSIFICATION *Continued*

        pNbiii   Extension of tumor beyond the capsule of a lymph node metastasis less than 2 cm in greatest dimension

        pN1biv   Metastasis to a lymph node 2 cm or more in greatest dimension

pN2   Metastasis to ipsilateral axillary lymph nodes that are fixed to one another or to other structures

pN3   Metastasis to ipsilateral internal mammary lymph node(s)

DISTANT METASTASIS (M)

MX   Distant metastasis cannot be assessed

M0   No distant metastasis

M1   Distant metastasis (includes metastasis to ipsilateral supraclavicular lymph node[s])

Stage Grouping

Stage 0	Tis	N0	M0
Stage I	T1*	N0	M0
Stage IIA	T0	N1	M0
	T1*	N1**	M0
	T2	N0	M0
Stage IIB	T2	N1	M0
	T3	N0	M0
Stage IIIA	T0	N2	M0
	T1*	N2	M0
	T2	N2	M0
	T3	N1	M0
	T3	N2	M0
Stage IIIB	T4	Any N	M0
	Any T	N3	M0
Stage IV	Any T	Any N	M1

* T1 includes T1mic.

** The prognosis of patients with N1a is similar to that of patients with pN0.

From **AJCC Cancer Staging Handbook.** *Philadelphia: Lippincott-Raven, 1998:162–163.*

CARCINOMA OF THE LACRIMAL GLAND CLASSIFICATION

PRIMARY TUMOR (T)

TX   Primary tumor cannot be assessed

T0   No evidence of primary tumor

T1   Tumor 2.5 cm or less in greatest dimension limited to the lacrimal gland

T2   Tumor 2.5 cm or less in greatest dimension invading the periosteum of the fossa of the lacrimal gland

T3   Tumor more than 2.5 cm but not more than 5 cm in greatest dimension

    T3a   Tumor limited to the lacrimal gland

    T3b   Tumor invades the periosteum of the fossa of the lacrimal gland

T4   Tumor more than 5 cm in greatest dimension

    T4a   Tumor invades the orbital soft tissues, optic nerve, or globe without bone invasion

    T4b   Tumor invades the orbital soft tissues, optic nerve, or globe with bone invasion

REGIONAL LYMPH NODES (N)

NX   Regional lymph nodes cannot be assessed

N0   No regional lymph node metastasis

N1   Regional lymph node metastasis

DISTANT METASTASIS (M)

MX   Distant metastasis cannot be assessed

M0   No distant metastasis

M1   Distant metastasis

Stage Grouping

No stage grouping presently is recommended.

From **AJCC Cancer Staging Handbook.** *Philadelphia: Lippincott-Raven, 1998:251–252.*

CARCINOMA OF THE SKIN CLASSIFICATIONS (EXCLUDING EYELID, VULVA, AND PENIS)

PRIMARY TUMOR (T)

TX	Primary tumor cannot be assessed
T0	No evidence of primary tumor
Tis	Carcinoma in situ
T1	Tumor 2 cm or less in greatest dimension
T2	Tumor more than 2 cm but not more than 5 cm in greatest dimension
T3	Tumor more than 5 cm in greatest dimension
T4	Tumor invades deep extradermal structures (i.e., cartilage, skeletal muscle, or bone)

REGIONAL LYMPH NODES (N)

NX	Regional lymph nodes cannot be assessed
N0	No regional lymph node metastasis
N1	Regional lymph node metastasis

DISTANT METASTASIS (M)

MX	Distant metastasis cannot be assessed
M0	No distant metastasis
M1	Distant metastasis

Stage Grouping

Stage 0	Tis	N0	M0
Stage I	T1	N0	M0
Stage II	T2	N0	M0
	T3	N0	M0
Stage III	T4	N0	M0
	Any T	N1	M0
Stage IV	Any T	Any N	M1

From AJCC Cancer Staging Handbook. Philadelphia: Lippincott-Raven, 1998:148–149.

CERVICAL (CERVIX UTERI) CANCER CLASSIFICATION

PRIMARY TUMOR (T)

TNM CATEGORIES	FIGO (Fédération Internationale de Gynécologie et d'Obstétrique) STAGES	
TX	—	Primary tumor cannot be assessed
T0	—	No evidence of primary tumor
Tis	—	Carcinoma in situ
T1	I	Cervical carcinoma confined to uterus (extension to corpus should be disregarded)
T1a	IA	Invasive carcinoma diagnosed only by microscopy. All macroscopically visible lesions—even with superficial invasion—are T1b/lB. Stromal invasion with a maximal depth of 5.0 mm measured from the base of the epithelium and a horizontal spread of 7.0 mm or less. Vascular space involvement, venous or lymphatic, does not affect classification.
T1a1	IA1	Measured stromal invasion 3.0 mm or less in depth and 7.0 mm or less in horizontal spread
T1a2	IA2	Measured stromal invasion more than 3.0 mm and not more than 5.0 mm with a horizontal spread 7.0 mm or less
T1b	IB	Clinically visible lesion confined to the cervix or microscopic lesion greater than T1a/IA2
T1b1	IB1	Clinically visible lesion 4.0 cm or less in greatest dimension
T1b2	IB2	Clinically visible lesion more than 4.0 cm in greatest dimension
T2	II	Cervical carcinoma invades beyond uterus but not to pelvic wall or to the lower third of vagina
T2a	IIA	Tumor without parametrial invasion
T2b	IIB	Tumor with parametrial invasion
T3	III	Tumor extends to the pelvic wall, and/or involves the lower third of the vagina, and/or causes hydronephrosis or nonfunctioning kidney
T3a	IIIA	Tumor involves lower third of the vagina, no extension to pelvic wall
T3b	IIIB	Tumor extends to pelvic wall and/or causes hydronephrosis or nonfunctioning kidney

Table continued on following page

CERVICAL (CERVIX UTERI) CANCER CLASSIFICATION *Continued*

PRIMARY TUMOR (T)

TNM CATEGORIES	FIGO (Fédération Internationale de Gynécologie et d'Obstétrique) STAGES	
T4	IVA	Tumor invades mucosa of the bladder or rectum, and/or extends beyond true pelvis (bullous edema is not sufficient to classify a tumor as T4)
M1	IVB	Distant metastasis

REGIONAL LYMPH NODES (N)

NX	Regional lymph nodes cannot be assessed
N0	No regional lymph node metastasis
N1	Regional lymph node metastasis

DISTANT METASTASIS (M)

MX	Distant metastasis cannot be assessed
M0	No distant metastasis
M1	Distant metastasis

pTNM Pathologic Classification

The pT, pN, and pM categories correspond to the T, N, and M categories.

Stage Grouping

Stage 0	Tis	N0	M0
Stage IA1	T1a1	N0	M0
Stage IA2	T1a2	N0	M0
Stage IB1	T1b1	N0	M0
Stage IB2	T1b2	N0	M0
Stage IIA	T12a	N0	M0
Stage IIB	T12b	N0	M0
Stage IIIA	T13a	N0	M0
Stage IIIB	T1	N1	M0
	T2	N1	M0
	T3a	N1	M0
	T3b	Any N	M0
Stage IVA	T4	Any N	M0
Stage IVB	Any T	Any N	M1

From AJCC Cancer Staging Handbook. Philadelphia: Lippincott-Raven, 1998:180–181.

COLON AND RECTUM CANCER CLASSIFICATION

PRIMARY TUMOR (T)

TX	Primary tumor cannot be assessed
T0	No evidence of primary tumor
Tis	Carcinoma in situ: Intraepithelial or invasion of lamina propria*
T1	Tumor invades submucosa
T2	Tumor invades muscularis propria
T3	Tumor invades through the muscularis propria into the subserosa, or into nonperitonealized pericolic or perirectal tissues
T4	Tumor directly invades other organs or structures, and/or perforates visceral peritoneum†

REGIONAL LYMPH NODES (N)

NX	Regional lymph nodes cannot be assessed
N0	No regional lymph node metastasis
N1	Metastasis in one to three regional lymph nodes
N2	Metastasis in four or more regional lymph nodes

DISTANT METASTASIS (M)

MX	Distant metastasis cannot be assessed
M0	No distant metastasis
M1	Distant metastasis

Stage Grouping

AJCC/UICC				DUKES‡
Stage 0	Tis	N0	M0	—
Stage I	T1	N0	M0	A
	T2	N0	M0	—
Stage II	T3	N0	M0	B
	T4	N0	M0	—
Stage III	Any T	N1	M0	C
	Any T	N2	M0	—
Stage IV	Any T	Any N	M1	D§

* Tis includes cancer cells confined within the glandular basement membrane (intraepithelial) or lamina propria (intramucosal) with no extension through the muscularis mucosae into the submucosa.

† Direct invasion in T4 includes invasion of other segments of the colorectum by way of the serosa; for example, invasion of the sigmoid colon by a carcinoma of the cecum.

‡ Dukes B is a composite of better (T3 N0 M0) and worse (T4 N0 M0) prognostic groups, as is Dukes C (any TN1 M0 and any TN2 M0).

§ Although not in the original scheme, a Dukes D classification is often used to signify metastatic disease.

*From **AJCC Cancer Staging Handbook**. Philadelphia: Lippincott-Raven, 1998:84–85.*

CONJUNCTIVA CANCER CLASSIFICATION

PRIMARY TUMOR (T)

TX	Primary tumor cannot be assessed
T0	No evidence of primary tumor
Tis	Carcinoma in situ
T1	Tumor 5 mm or less in greatest dimension
T2	Tumor more than 5 mm in greatest dimension, without invasion of adjacent structures
T3	Tumor invades adjacent structures, excluding the orbit
T4	Tumor invades the orbit

REGIONAL LYMPH NODES (N)

NX	Regional lymph nodes cannot be assessed
N0	No regional lymph node metastasis
N1	Regional lymph node metastasis

DISTANT METASTASIS (M)

MX	Distant metastasis cannot be assessed
M0	No distant metastasis
M1	Distant Metastasis

Stage Grouping

No stage grouping presently is recommended.

From **AJCC Cancer Staging Handbook.** *Philadelphia: Lippincott-Raven, 1998:235–236.*

UTERUS (CORPUS UTERI) CANCER CLASSIFICATION

PRIMARY TUMOR (T)

TNM CATEGORIES		FIGO STAGES	
TX			Primary tumor cannot be assessed
T0			No evidence of primary tumor
Tis			Carcinoma in situ
T1		I	Tumor confined to corpus uteri
	T1a	IA	Tumor limited to endometrium
	T1b	IB	Tumor invades up to or less than one half of the myometrium
	T1c	IC	Tumor invades to more than one half of the myometrium
T2		II	Tumor invades cervix but does not extend beyond uterus
	T2a	IIA	Endocervical glandular involvement only
	T2b	IIB	Cervical stromal invasion
T3		III	Local and/or regional spread as specified in T3a, b, and/or N1 and FIGO IIIA, B, and C below

UTERUS (CORPUS UTERI) CANCER CLASSIFICATION *Continued*

PRIMARY TUMOR (T)

TNM CATEGORIES	**FIGO STAGES**	
T3a	IIIA	Tumor involves serosa and/or adnexa (direct extension or metastasis) and/or cancer cells in ascites or peritoneal washings
T3b	IIIB	Vaginal involvement (direct extension or metastasis)
N1	IIIC	Metastasis to the pelvic and/or paraaortic lymph nodes
T4	IVA	Tumor invades bladder mucosa and/or bowel mucosa (bullous edema is not sufficient to classify a tumor as T4)
M1	IVB	Distant metastasis. (Excluding metastasis to vagina, pelvic serosa, or adnexa; including metastasis to intra-abdominal lymph nodes other than paraaortic, and/or inguinal lymph nodes.)

REGIONAL LYMPH NODES (N)

NX	Regional lymph nodes cannot be assessed
N0	No regional lymph node metastasis
N1	Regional lymph node metastasis

DISTANT METASTASIS (M)

MX	Distant metastasis cannot be assessed
M0	No distant metastasis
M1	Distant metastasis

pTNM PATHOLOGIC CLASSIFICATION

The pT, pN, and pM categories correspond to the T, N, and M categories.

Stage Grouping

Stage 0	Tis	N0	M0
Stage IA	T1a	N0	M0
Stage IB	T1b	N0	M0
Stage IC	T1c	N0	M0
Stage IIA	T2a	N0	M0
Stage IIB	T2b	N0	M0
Stage IIIA	T3a	N0	M0
Stage IIIB	T3b	N0	M0
Stage IIIC	T1	N1	M0
	T2	N1	M0
	T3a	N1	M0
	T3b	N1	M0
Stage IVA	T4	Any N	M0
Stage IVB	Any T	Any N	M1

From **AJCC Cancer Staging Handbook.** *Philadelphia: Lippincott-Raven, 1998:184–185.*

ESOPHAGUS CANCER CLASSIFICATION

PRIMARY TUMOR (T)

TX	Primary tumor cannot be assessed
T0	No evidence of primary tumor
Tis	Carcinoma in situ
T1	Tumor invades lamina propria or submucosa
T2	Tumor invades muscularis propria
T3	Tumor invades adventitia
T4	Tumor invades adjacent structures

REGIONAL LYMPH NODES (N)

NX	Regional lymph nodes cannot be assessed
N0	No regional lymph node metastasis
N1	Regional lymph node metastasis

DISTANT METASTASIS (M)

MX	Distant metastasis cannot be assessed
M0	No distant metastasis
M1	Distant metastasis

Tumors of the lower thoracic esophagus:
- M1a   Metastasis in celiac lymph nodes
- M1b   Other distant metastasis

Tumors of the midthoracic esophagus:
- M1a   Not applicable
- M1b   Nonregional lymph nodes and/or other distant metastasis

Tumors or the upper thoracic esophagus:
- M1a   Metastasis in cervical nodes
- M1b   Other distant metastasis

Stage Grouping

Stage 0	Tis	N0	M0
Stage I	T1	N0	M0
Stage IIA	T2	N0	M0
	T3	N0	M0
Stage IIB	T1	N1	M0
	T2	N1	M0
Stage III	T3	N1	M0
	T4	Any N	M0
Stage IV	Any T	Any N	M1
Stage IVA	Any T	Any N	M1a
Stage IVB	Any T	Any N	M1b

From AJCC Cancer Staging Handbook. Philadelphia: Lippincott-Raven, 1998:67.

EXOCRINE PANCREAS CANCER CLASSIFICATION

PRIMARY TUMOR (T)

TX	Primary tumor cannot be assessed
T0	No evidence of primary tumor
Tis	In situ carcinoma
T1	Tumor limited to the pancreas 2 cm or less in greatest dimension
T2	Tumor limited to the pancreas more than 2 cm in greatest dimension
T3	Tumor extends directly into any of the following: duodenum, bile duct, peripancreatic tissues
T4	Tumor extends directly into any of the following: stomach, spleen, colon, adjacent large vessels

REGIONAL LYMPH NODES (N)

NX	Regional lymph nodes cannot be assessed
N0	No regional lymph node metastasis
N1	Regional lymph node metastasis
	pN1a Metastasis in a single regional lymph node
	pN1b Metastasis in multiple regional lymph nodes

DISTANT METASTASIS (M)

MX	Distant metastasis cannot be assessed
M0	No distant metastasis
M1	Distant metastasis

Stage Grouping

Stage 0	Tis	N0	M0
Stage I	T1	N0	M0
	T2	N0	M0
Stage II	T3	N0	M0
Stage III	T1	N1	M0
	T2	N1	M0
	T3	N1	M0
Stage IVA	T4	Any N	M0
Stage IVB	Any T	Any N	M1

From **AJCC Cancer Staging Handbook.** *Philadelphia: Lippincott-Raven, 1998:112–113.*

EXTRAHEPATIC BILE DUCTS CANCER CLASSIFICATION

PRIMARY TUMOR (T)

TX   Primary tumor cannot be assessed
T0   No evidence of primary tumor
Tis   Carcinoma in situ
T1   Tumor invades subepithelial connective tissue or fibromuscular layer
      T1a   Tumor invades subepithelial connective tissue
      T1b   Tumor invades fibromuscular layer
T2   Tumor invades perifibromuscular connective tissue
T3   Tumor invades adjacent structures: liver, pancreas, duodenum, gallbladder, colon, stomach

REGIONAL LYMPH NODES (N)

NX   Regional lymph nodes cannot be assessed
N0   No regional lymph node metastasis
N1   Metastasis in cystic duct, pericholedochal and/or hilar lymph nodes (i.e., in the hepatoduodenal ligament)
N2   Metastasis in peripancreatic (head only), periduodenal, periportal, celiac, and/or superior mesenteric and/or posterior pancreaticoduodenal lymph nodes

DISTANT METASTASIS (M)

MX   Distant metastasis cannot be assessed
M0   No distant metastasis
M1   Distant metastasis

Stage Grouping

Stage 0	Tis	N0	M0
Stage I	T1	N0	M0
Stage II	T2	N0	M0
Stage III	T1	N1	M0
	T1	N2	M0
	T2	N1	M0
	T2	N2	M0
Stage IVA	T3	Any N	M0
Stage IVB	Any T	Any N	M1

From **AJCC Cancer Staging Handbook.** *Philadelphia: Lippincott-Raven, 1998:102–103.*

EYELID CANCER CLASSIFICATION

PRIMARY TUMOR (T)

TX	Primary tumor cannot be assessed
T0	No evidence of primary tumor
Tis	Carcinoma in situ
T1	Tumor of any size, not invading the tarsal plate or, at the eyelid margin, 5 mm or less in greatest dimension
T2	Tumor invades tarsal plate or, at the eyelid margin, more than 5 mm but not more than 10 mm in greatest dimension
T3	Tumor involves full eyelid thickness or, at the eyelid margin, more than 10 mm in greatest dimension
T4	Tumor invades adjacent structures

REGIONAL LYMPH NODES (N)

NX	Regional lymph nodes cannot be assessed
N0	No regional lymph node metastasis
N1	Regional lymph node metastasis

DISTANT METASTASIS (M)

MX	Distant metastasis cannot be assessed
M0	No distant metastasis
M1	Distant metastasis

Stage Grouping

No stage grouping presently is recommended.

From AJCC Cancer Staging Handbook. Philadelphia: Lippincott-Raven, 1998:232.

FALLOPIAN TUBE CANCER CLASSIFICATION

PRIMARY TUMOR (T)

TNM CATEGORIES		FIGO STAGES	
TX			Primary tumor cannot be assessed
T0			No evidence of primary tumor
Tis		0	Carcinoma in situ (limited to tubal mucosa)
T1		I	Tumor limited to the fallopian tube(s)
	T1a	IA	Tumor limited to one tube, without penetrating the serosal surface; no ascites
	T1b	IB	Tumor limited to both tubes, without penetrating the serosal surface; no ascites
	T1c	IC	Tumor limited to one or both tubes with extension onto or through the tubal serosa, or with malignant cells in ascites or peritoneal washings

Table continued on following page

FALLOPIAN TUBE CANCER CLASSIFICATION *Continued*

PRIMARY TUMOR (T)

TNM CATEGORIES	FIGO STAGES	
T2	II	Tumor involves one or both fallopian tubes with pelvic extension
T2a	IIA	Extension and/or metastasis to the uterus and/or ovaries
T2b	IIB	Extension to other pelvic structures
T2c	IIC	Pelvic extension with malignant cells in ascites or peritoneal washings
T3 and/or N1	III	Tumor involves one or both fallopian tubes, with peritoneal implants outside the pelvis and/or positive regional lymph nodes
T3a	IIIA	Microscopic peritoneal metastasis outside the pelvis
T3b	IIIB	Macroscopic peritoneal metastasis outside the pelvis 2 cm or less in greatest dimension
T3c and/or N1	IIIC	Peritoneal metastasis more than 2 cm in diameter and/or positive regional lymph nodes
M1	IV	Distant metastases (excludes peritoneal metastasis)

REGIONAL LYMPH NODES (N)

NX	Regional lymph nodes cannot be assessed
N0	No regional lymph node metastasis
N1	Regional lymph node metastasis

DISTANT METASTASIS (M)

MX	Distant metastasis cannot be assessed
M0	No distant metastasis
M1	Distant metastasis

Stage Grouping

Stage 0	Tis	N0	M0
Stage IA	T1a	N0	M0
Stage IB	T1b	N0	M0
Stage IC	T1c	N0	M0
Stage IIA	T2a	N0	M0
Stage IIB	T2b	N0	M0
Stage IIC	T2c	N0	M0
Stage IIIA	T3a	N0	M0
Stage IIIB	T3b	N0	M0
Stage IIIC	T3c	N0	M0
	Any T	N1	M0
Stage IV	Any T	Any N	M1

From AJCC Cancer Staging Handbook. Philadelphia: Lippincott-Raven, 1998:191–192.

GALLBLADDER CANCER CLASSIFICATION

PRIMARY TUMOR (T)

TX	Primary tumor cannot be assessed
T0	No evidence of primary tumor
Tis	Carcinoma in situ
T1	Tumor invades lamina propria or muscle layer
	T1a Tumor invades lamina propria
	T1b Tumor invades muscle layer
T2	Tumor invades perimuscular connective tissue; no extension beyond serosa or into liver
T3	Tumor perforates the serosa (visceral peritoneum) or directly invades one adjacent organ, or both (extension 2 cm or less into liver)
T4	Tumor extends more than 2 cm into liver, and/or into two or more adjacent organs (stomach, duodenum, colon, pancreas, omentum, extrahepatic bile ducts, and involvement of liver)

REGIONAL LYMPH NODES (N)

NX	Regional lymph nodes cannot be assessed
N0	No regional lymph node metastasis
N1	Metastasis in cystic duct, pericholedochal, and/or hilar lymph nodes (i.e., in the hepatoduodenal ligament)
N2	Metastasis in peripancreatic (head only), periduodenal, periportal, celiac, and/or superior mesenteric lymph nodes

DISTANT METASTASIS (M)

MX	Distant metastasis cannot be assessed
M0	No distant metastasis
M1	Distant metastasis

Stage Grouping

Stage 0	Tis	N0	M0
Stage I	T1	N0	M0
Stage II	T2	N0	M0
Stage III	T1	N1	M0
	T2	N1	M0
	T3	N0	M0
	T3	N1	M0
Stage IVA	T4	N0	M0
	T4	N1	M0
Stage IVB	Any T	N2	M0
	Any T	Any N	M1

From **AJCC Cancer Staging Handbook.** *Philadelphia: Lippincott-Raven, 1998:98–99.*

GESTATIONAL TROPHOBLASTIC TUMOR CANCER CLASSIFICATION

PRIMARY TUMOR (T)

TX	Primary tumor cannot be assessed
T0	No evidence of primary tumor
T1	Disease limited to uterus
T2	Disease outside of uterus but is limited to genital structures (ovary, tube, vagina, broad ligaments)

DISTANT METASTASIS (M)

M0	No clinical metastasis
M1a	Lung metastasis
M1b	All other distant metastasis

RISK FACTORS

1. hCG >100,000 IU/24-hour urine
2. The detection of disease more than six months from termination of the antecedent pregnancy

Stage Grouping

STAGE	T	M	RISK FACTORS
IA	T1	M0	Without
IB	T1	M0	One
IC	T1	M0	Two
IIA	T2	M0	Without
IIB	T2	M0	One
IIC	T2	M0	Two
IIIA	Any T	M1a	Without
IIIB	Any T	M1a	One
IIIC	Any T	M1a	Two
IVA	Any T	M1b	Without
IVB	Any T	M1b	One
IVC	Any T	M1b	Two

*From **AJCC Cancer Staging Handbook**. Philadelphia: Lippincott-Raven, 1998:195–196.*

HODGKIN'S DISEASE (LYMPHOMA) CLASSIFICATION
Stage Grouping

Stage I   Involvement of a single lymph node region (I) or localized involvement of a single extralymphatic organ or site (I_E).

Stage II   Involvement of two or more lymph node regions on the same side of the diaphragm (II) or localized involvement of a single associated extralymphatic organ or site and its regional lymph node(s) with or without involvement of other lymph node regions on the same side of the diaphragm (II_E).

Stage III   Involvement of lymph node regions on both sides of the diaphragm (III), which also may be accompanied by localized involvement of an associated extralymphatic organ or site (III_E), by involvement of the spleen (III_S), or both (III_{E+S}).

Stage IV   Disseminated (multifocal) involvement of one or more extralymphatic organs, with or without associated lymph node involvement, or isolated extralymphatic organ involvement with distant (nonregional) nodal involvement.

Note: The number of lymph node regions involved may be indicated by a subscript (e.g., II_3).

SYSTEMIC SYMPTOMS
Each stage is subdivided into A or B categories, B for those with defined systemic symptoms and A for those without. B patients have unexplained weight loss (more than 10% of body weight in the past 6 months), unexplained fever with temperatures above 38°C, and drenching night sweats. Pruritus usually does not qualify for B classification.

From AJCC Cancer Staging Handbook. *Philadelphia: Lippincott-Raven, 1998:259–260.*

KIDNEY CANCER CLASSIFICATION

This classification applies only to the renal cell cancers.

PRIMARY TUMOR (T)

TX	Primary tumor cannot be assessed
T0	No evidence of primary tumor
T1	Tumor 7 cm or less in greatest dimension limited to the kidney
T2	Tumor more than 7 cm in greatest dimension limited to the kidney
T3	Tumor extends into major veins or invades the adrenal gland or perinephric tissues, but not beyond Gerota's fascia

T3a   Tumor invades the adrenal gland or perinephric tissues but not beyond Gerota's fascia

T3b   Tumor grossly extends into the renal vein(s) or vena cava below the diaphragm

T3c   Tumor grossly extends into the renal vein(s) or vena cava above the diaphragm

T4	Tumor invades beyond Gerota's fascia

REGIONAL LYMPH NODES (N)*

NX	Regional lymph nodes cannot be assessed
N0	No regional lymph node metastases
N1	Metastasis in a single regional lymph node
N2	Metastasis in more than one regional lymph node

DISTANT METASTASIS (M)

MX	Distant metastasis cannot be assessed
M0	No distant metastasis
M1	Distant metastasis

Stage Grouping

Stage I	T1	N0	M0
Stage II	T2	N0	M0
Stage III	T1	N1	M0
	T2	N1	M0
	T3a	N0	M0
	T3a	N1	M0
	T3b	N0	M0
	T3b	N1	M0
	T3c	N0	M0
	T3c	N1	M0
Stage IV	T4	N0	M0
	T4	N1	M0
	Any T	N2	M0
	Any T	Any N	M1

* Laterality does not affect the N classification.

From AJCC Cancer Staging Handbook. *Philadelphia: Lippincott-Raven, 1998:216.*

LARYNX CANCER CLASSIFICATION

PRIMARY TUMOR (T)

TX   Primary tumor cannot be assessed
T0   No evidence of primary tumor
Tis   Carcinoma in situ

Supraglottis

T1   Tumor limited to one subsite of supraglottis with normal vocal cord mobility
T2   Tumor invades mucosa of more than one adjacent subsite of supraglottis or glottis or region outside the supraglottis (e.g., mucosa of base of tongue, vallecula, medial wall of pyriform sinus) without fixation of the larynx
T3   Tumor limited to larynx with vocal cord fixation and/or invades any of the following: postcricoid area, preepiglottic tissues
T4   Tumor invades through the thyroid cartilage, and/or extends into soft tissues of the neck, thyroid, and/or esophagus

Glottis

T1   Tumor limited to the vocal cord(s) (may involve anterior or posterior commissure) with normal mobility
        T1a   Tumor limited to one vocal cord
        T1b   Tumor involves both vocal cords
T2   Tumor extends to supraglottis and/or subglottis, and/or with impaired vocal cord mobility
T3   Tumor limited to the larynx with vocal cord fixation
T4   Tumor invades through the thyroid cartilage and/or to other tissues beyond the larynx (e.g., trachea, soft tissues of neck, including thyroid, pharynx)

Subglottis

T1   Tumor limited to the subglottis
T2   Tumor extends to vocal cord(s) with normal or impaired mobility
T3   Tumor limited to larynx with vocal cord fixation
T4   Tumor invades through cricoid or thyroid cartilage and/or extends to other tissues beyond the larynx (e.g., trachea, soft tissues of neck, including thyroid, esophagus)

REGIONAL LYMPH NODES (N)

NX   Regional lymph nodes cannot be assessed
N0   No regional lymph node metastasis
N1   Metastasis in a single ipsilateral lymph node, 3 cm or less in greatest dimension
N2   Metastasis in a single ipsilateral lymph node, more than 3 cm but not more than 6 cm in greatest dimension, or in multiple ipsilateral lymph nodes, none more than 6 cm in greatest dimension, or in bilateral or contralateral lymph nodes, none more than 6 cm in greatest dimension
        N2a   Metastasis in a single ipsilateral lymph node more than 3 cm but not more than 6 cm in greatest dimension

Table continued on following page

LARYNX CANCER CLASSIFICATION *Continued*

N2b   Metastasis in multiple ipsilateral lymph nodes, none more than 6 cm in greatest dimension

N2c   Metastasis in bilateral or contralateral lymph nodes, none more than 6 cm in greatest dimension

N3   Metastasis in a lymph node more than 6 cm in greatest dimension

DISTANT METASTASIS (M)

MX   Distant metastasis cannot be assessed

M0   No distant metastasis

M1   Distant metastasis

Stage Grouping

Stage 0	Tis	N0	M0
Stage I	T1	N0	M0
Stage II	T2	N0	M0
Stage III	T3	N0	M0
	T1	N1	M0
	T2	N1	M0
	T3	N1	M0
Stage IVA	T4	N0	M0
	T4	N1	M0
	Any T	N2	M0
Stage IVB	Any T	N3	M0
Stage IVC	Any T	Any N	M1

From AJCC Cancer Staging Handbook. Philadelphia: Lippincott-Raven, 1998:47–48.

LIP AND ORAL CAVITY CANCER CLASSIFICATION

PRIMARY TUMOR (T)

TX	Primary tumor cannot be assessed
T0	No evidence of primary tumor
Tis	Carcinoma in situ
T1	Tumor 2 cm or less in greatest dimension
T2	Tumor more than 2 cm but not more than 4 cm in greatest dimension
T3	Tumor more than 4 cm in greatest dimension
T4 (lip)	Tumor invades adjacent structures (e.g., through cortical bone, inferior alveolar nerve, floor of mouth, skin of face)
T4 (oral cavity)	Tumor invades adjacent structures (e.g., through cortical bone, into deep [extrinsic] muscle of tongue, maxillary sinus, skin; superficial erosion alone of bone/tooth socket by gingival primary is not sufficient to classify as T4

LIP AND ORAL CAVITY CANCER CLASSIFICATION *Continued*

REGIONAL LYMPH NODES (N)

NX   Regional lymph nodes cannot be assessed

N0   No regional lymph node metastasis

N1   Metastasis in a single ipsilateral lymph node, 3 cm or less in greatest dimension

N2   Metastasis in a single ipsilateral lymph node, more than 3 cm but not more than 6 cm in greatest dimension; or in multiple ipsilateral lymph nodes, none more than 6 cm in greatest dimension; or in bilateral or contralateral lymph nodes, none more than 6 cm in greatest dimension

     N2a   Metastasis in single ipsilateral lymph node more than 3 cm but not more than 6 cm in greatest dimension

     N2b   Metastasis in multiple ipsilateral lymph nodes, none more than 6 cm in greatest dimension

     N2c   Metastasis in bilateral or contralateral lymph nodes, none more than 6 cm in greatest dimension

N3   Metastasis in a lymph node more than 6 cm in greatest dimension

DISTANT METASTASIS (M)

MX   Distant metastasis cannot be assessed

M0   No distant metastasis

M1   Distant metastasis

Stage Grouping

Stage 0	Tis	N0	M0
Stage I	T1	N0	M0
Stage II	T2	N0	M0
Stage III	T3	N0	M0
	T1	N1	M0
	T2	N1	M0
	T3	N1	M0
Stage IVA	T4	N0	M0
	T4	N1	M0
	Any T	N2	M0
Stage IVB	Any T	N3	M0
Stage IVC	Any T	Any N	M1

*From **AJCC Cancer Staging Handbook**. Philadelphia: Lippincott-Raven, 1998:31–32.*

LIVER CANCER CLASSIFICATION

PRIMARY TUMOR (T)

TX	Primary tumor cannot be assessed
T0	No evidence of primary tumor
T1	Solitary tumor 2 cm or less in greatest dimension without vascular invasion
T2	Solitary tumor 2 cm or less in greatest dimension with vascular invasion, or multiple tumors limited to one lobe, none more than 2 cm in greatest dimension without vascular invasion
T3	Solitary tumor more than 2 cm in greatest dimension with vascular invasion, or multiple tumors limited to one lobe, none more than 2 cm in greatest dimension, with vascular invasion, or multiple tumors limited to one lobe, any more than 2 cm in greatest dimension, with or without vascular invasion
T4	Multiple tumors in more than one lobe or tumor(s) involve(s) a major branch of the portal or hepatic vein(s) or invasion of adjacent organs other than the gallbladder or perforation of the visceral peritoneum

REGIONAL LYMPH (N)

NX	Regional lymph nodes cannot be assessed
N0	No regional lymph node metastasis
N1	Regional lymph node metastasis

DISTANT METASTASIS (M)

MX	Distant metastasis cannot be assessed
M0	No distant metastasis
M1	Distant metastasis

Stage Grouping

Stage I	T1	N0	M0
Stage II	T2	N0	M0
Stage IIIA	T3	N0	M0
Stage IIIB	T1	N1	M0
	T2	N1	M0
	T3	N1	M0
Stage IVA	T4	Any N	M0
Stage IVB	Any T	Any N	M1

From AJCC Cancer Staging Handbook. Philadelphia: Lippincott-Raven, 1998:94–95.

LUNG CANCER CLASSIFICATION

PRIMARY TUMOR (T)

TX   Primary tumor cannot be assessed, or tumor proven by the presence of malignant cells in sputum or bronchial washings but not visualized by imaging or bronchoscopy

T0   No evidence of primary tumor

Tis   Carcinoma in situ

T1   Tumor 3 cm or less in greatest dimension, surrounded by lung or visceral pleura, without bronchoscopic evidence of invasion more proximal than the lobar bronchus* (i.e., not in the main bronchus)

T2   Tumor with any of the following features of size or extent:
More than 3 cm in greatest dimension
Involves main bronchus, 2 cm or more distal to the carina
Invades the visceral pleura
Associated with atelectasis or obstructive pneumonitis that extends to the hilar region but does not involve the entire lung

T3   Tumor of any size that directly invades any of the following: chest wall, diaphragm, mediastinal pleura, parietal pericardium; or tumor in the main bronchus less than 2 cm distal to the carina, but without involvement of the carina; or associated atelectasis or obstructive pneumonitis of the entire lung

T4   Tumor of any size that invades any of the following: mediastinum, heart, great vessels, trachea, esophagus, vertebral body, carina; or separate tumor nodules in the same lobe; or tumor with a malignant pleural effusion**

REGIONAL LYMPH NODES (N)

NX   Regional lymph nodes cannot be assessed

N0   No regional lymph node metastasis

N1   Metastasis to ipsilateral peribronchial and/or ipsilateral hilar lymph nodes, and intrapulmonary nodes including involvement by direct extension of the primary tumor

N2   Metastasis to ipsilateral mediastinal and/or subcarinal lymph node(s)

N3   Metastasis to contralateral mediastinal, contralateral hilar, ipsilateral or contralateral scalene, or supraclavicular lymph node(s)

DISTANT METASTASIS (M)

MX   Distant metastasis cannot be assessed

M0   No distant metastasis

M1   Distant metastasis present

Stage Grouping

Stage grouping of the TNM subsets has been revised as follows:

Occult Carcinoma	TX	N0	M0
Stage 0	Tis	N0	M0
Stage IA	T1	N0	M0
Stage IB	T2	N0	M0

Table continued on following page

LUNG CANCER CLASSIFICATION *Continued*

Stage IIA	T1	N1	M0
Stage IIB	T2	N1	M0
	T3	N0	M0
Stage IIIA	T1	N2	M0
	T2	N2	M0
	T3	N1	M0
	T3	N2	M0
Stage IIIB	Any T	N3	M0
	T4	Any N	M0
Stage IV	Any T	Any N	M1

* The uncommon superficial tumor of any size with its invasive component limited to the bronchial wall, which may extend proximal to the main bronchus, also is classified T1.

** Most pleural effusions associated with lung cancer are due to tumor. However, there are a few patients in whom multiple cytopathologic examinations of pleural fluid are negative for tumor. In these cases, fluid is nonbloody and is not an exudate. When these elements and clinical judgment dictate that the effusion is not related to the tumor, the effusion should be excluded as a staging element and the patient should be staged T1, T2, or T3.

From AJCC Cancer Staging Handbook. **Philadelphia: Lippincott-Raven, 1998:122–123.**

MAJOR SALIVARY GLANDS CANCER CLASSIFICATION

PRIMARY TUMOR (T)

TX	Primary tumor cannot be assessed
T0	No evidence of primary tumor
T1	Tumor 2 cm or less in greatest dimension without extraparenchymal extension
T2	Tumor more than 2 cm but not more than 4 cm in greatest dimension without extraparenchymal extension
T3	Tumor having extraparenchymal extension without seventh nerve involvement and/or more than 4 cm but not more than 6 cm in greatest dimension
T4	Tumor invades base of skull, seventh nerve, and/or exceeds 6 cm in greatest dimension

REGIONAL LYMPH NODES (N)

NX	Regional lymph nodes cannot be assessed
N0	No regional lymph node metastasis
N1	Metastasis in a single ipsilateral lymph node, 3 cm or less in greatest dimension
N2	Metastasis in a single ipsilateral lymph node, more than 3 cm but not more than 6 cm in greatest dimension, or in bilateral or contralateral lymph nodes, none more than 6 cm in greatest dimension

DISTANT METASTASIS (M)

MX	Distant metastasis cannot be assessed
M0	No distant metastasis
M1	Distant metastasis

Stage Grouping

Stage I	T1	N0	M0
	T2	N0	M0
Stage II	T3	N0	M0
Stage III	T1	N1	M0
	T2	N1	M0
Stage IV	T4	N0	M0
	T3	N1	M0
	T4	N1	M0
	Any T	N2	M0
	Any T	N3	M0
	Any T	Any N	M1

*From **AJCC Cancer Staging Handbook**. Philadelphia: Lippincott-Raven, 1998:58–59.*

MALIGNANT MELANOMA OF THE CONJUNCTIVA CLASSIFICATION

PRIMARY TUMOR (T)

TX	Primary tumor cannot be assessed
T0	No evidence of primary tumor
T1	Tumor(s) of bulbar conjunctiva occupying one quadrant or less
T2	Tumor(s) of bulbar conjunctiva occupying more than one quadrant
T3	Tumor(s) of conjunctival fornix and/or palpebral conjunctiva and/or caruncle
T4	Tumor invades eyelid, cornea, and/or orbit

REGIONAL LYMPH NODES (N)

NX	Regional lymph nodes cannot be assessed
N0	No regional lymph node metastasis
N1	Regional lymph node metastasis

DISTANT METASTASIS (M)

MX	Distant metastasis cannot be assessed
M0	No distant metastasis
M1	Distant metastasis

PATHOLOGIC CLASSIFICATION (pTNM)

Primary Tumor (pT)

pTX	Primary tumor cannot be assessed
pT0	No evidence of primary tumor
pT1	Tumor(s) of bulbar conjunctiva occupying one quadrant or less and 2 mm or less in thickness
pT2	Tumor(s) of bulbar conjunctiva occupying more than one quadrant and 2 mm or less in thickness
pT3	Tumor(s) of the conjunctival fornix and/or palpebral conjunctiva and/or caruncle or tumor(s) of the bulbar conjunctiva, more than 2 mm in thickness
pT4	Tumor invades eyelid, cornea, and/or orbit

Regional Lymph Nodes (pN)

pNX	Regional lymph nodes cannot be assessed
pN0	No regional lymph node metastasis
pN1	Regional lymph node metastasis

Distant Metastasis (pM)

pMX	Distant metastasis cannot be assessed
pM0	No distant metastasis
pM1	Distant metastasis

Stage Grouping

No stage grouping presently is recommended.

From AJCC Cancer Staging Handbook. Philadelphia: Lippincott-Raven, 1998:237–238.

PRIMARY TUMOR (pT)

pTX Primary tumor cannot be assessed

pT0 No evidence of primary tumor

pTis Melanoma in situ (atypical melanocytic hyperplasia, severe melanocytic dysplasia), not an invasive malignant lesion (Clark's Level I)

pT1 Tumor 0.75 mm or less in thickness and invades the papillary dermis (Clark's Level II)

pT2 Tumor more than 0.75 mm but not more than 1.5 mm in thickness and/or invades to papillary-reticular dermal interface (Clark's Level III)

pT3 Tumor more than 1.5 mm but not more than 4 mm in thickness and/or invades the reticular dermis (Clark's Level IV)

   pT3a Tumor more than 1.5 mm but not more than 3 mm in thickness

   pT3b Tumor more than 3 mm but not more than 4 mm in thickness

pT4 Tumor more than 4 mm in thickness and/or invades the subcutaneous tissue (Clark's Level V) and/or satellite(s) within 2 cm of the primary tumor

   pT4a Tumor more than 4 mm in thickness and/or invades the subcutaneous tissue

   pT4b Satellite(s) within 2 cm of the primary tumor

REGIONAL LYMPH NODES (N)

NX Regional lymph nodes cannot be assessed

N0 No regional lymph node metastasis

N1 Metastasis 3 cm or less in greatest dimension in any regional lymph node(s)

N2 Metastasis more than 3 cm in greatest dimension in any regional lymph node(s) and/or in-transit metastasis

   N2a Metastasis more than 3 cm in greatest dimension in any regional lymph node(s)

   N2b In-transit metastasis

   N2c Both (N2a and N2b)

DISTANT METASTASIS (M)

MX Distant metastasis cannot be assessed

M0 No distant metastasis

M1 Distant metastasis

   M1a Metastasis in skin or subcutaneous tissue or lymph node(s) beyond the regional lymph nodes

   M1b Visceral metastasis

Stage Grouping

Stage 0	pTis	N0	M0
Stage I	pT1	N0	M0
	pT2	N0	M0
Stage II	pT3	N0	M0
Stage III	pT4	N0	M0
	Any pT	N1	M0
	Any pT	N2	M0
Stage IV	Any pT	Any N	M1

*From **AJCC Cancer Staging Handbook**. Philadelphia: Lippincott-Raven, 1998:157–158.*

MALIGNANT MELANOMA OF THE UVEA CLASSIFICATION

ANATOMIC SITES
Iris
Ciliary body
Choroid

IRIS

Primary Tumor (T)
TX   Primary tumor cannot be assessed
T0   No evidence of primary tumor
T1   Tumor limited to the iris
T2   Tumor involves one quadrant or less, with invasion into the anterior chamber angle
T3   Tumor involves more than one quadrant, with invasion into the anterior chamber angle, ciliary body, and/or choroid
T4   Tumor with extraocular extension

Regional Lymph Nodes (N)
NX   Regional lymph nodes cannot be assessed
N0   No regional lymph node metastasis
N1   Regional lymph node metastasis

Distant Metastasis (M)
MX   Distant metastasis cannot be assessed
M0   No distant metastasis
M1   Distant metastasis

CILIARY BODY

Primary Tumor (T)
TX   Primary tumor cannot be assessed
T0   No evidence of primary tumor
T1   Tumor limited to the ciliary body
T2   Tumor invades into anterior chamber and/or iris
T3   Tumor invades choroid
T4   Tumor with extraocular extension

Regional Lymph Nodes (N)
NX   Regional lymph nodes cannot be assessed
N0   No regional lymph node metastasis
N1   Regional lymph node metastasis

Distant Metastasis (M)
MX   Distant metastasis cannot be assessed
M0   No distant metastasis
M1   Distant metastasis

CHOROID

Primary Tumor (T)
TX   Primary tumor cannot be assessed
T0   No evidence of primary tumor
T1*   Tumor 10 mm or less in greatest dimension with an elevation 3 mm or less

MALIGNANT MELANOMA OF THE UVEA
CLASSIFICATION *Continued*

T1a   Tumor 7 mm or less in greatest dimension with an elevation 2 mm or less

T1b   Tumor more than 7 mm but not more than 10 mm in greatest dimension with an elevation more than 2 mm but not more than 3 mm

T2*   Tumor more than 10 mm but not more than 15 mm in greatest dimension with an elevation of more than 3 mm but not more than 5 mm

T3*   Tumor more than 15 mm in greatest dimension or with an elevation more than 5 mm

T4   Tumor with extraocular extension

Regional Lymph Nodes (N)

NX   Regional lymph nodes cannot be assessed

N0   No regional lymph node metastasis

N1   Regional lymph node metastasis

Distant Metastasis (M)

MX   Distant metastasis cannot be assessed

M0   No distant metastasis

M1   Distant metastasis

Stage Grouping

The classification of the structure most affected is used when more than one of the uveal structures is involved by tumor.

Iris and Ciliary Body

Stage I	T1	N0	M0
Stage II	T2	N0	M0
Stage III	T3	N0	M0
Stage IVA	T4	N0	M0
Stage IVB	Any T	N1	M0
	Any T	Any N	M1

Choroid

Stage IA	T1a	N0	M0
Stage IB	T1b	N0	M0
Stage II	T2	N0	M0
Stage III	T3	N0	M0
Stage IVA	T4	N0	M0
Stage IVB	Any T	N1	M0
	Any T	Any N	M1

* In clinical practice the tumor base may be estimated in optic disc diameters (dd) (average: 1 dd = 1.5 mm). The elevation may be estimated in optic diopters (average: 3 diopters = 1 mm). Other techniques used, such as ultrasonography and computerized stereometry, may provide a more accurate measurement.

From AJCC Cancer Staging Handbook. *Philadelphia: Lippincott-Raven, 1998:242–244.*

NON-HODGKIN'S LYMPHOMA CLASSIFICATION
Stage Grouping

Stage I	Involvement of a single lymph node region (I) or localized involvement of a single extralymphatic organ or site (I_E).
Stage II	Involvement of two or more lymph node regions on the same side of the diaphragm (II), or localized involvement of a single associated extralymphatic organ or site and its regional nodes with or without other lymph node regions on the same side of the diaphragm (II_E).
Stage III	Involvement of lymph node regions on both sides of the diaphragm (III), which also may be accompanied by localized involvement of an extralymphatic organ or site (III_E), by involvement of the spleen (III_S), or both ($III_{E + S}$).
Stage IV	Disseminated (multifocal) involvement of one or more extralymphatic organs, with or without associated lymph node involvement, or isolated extralymphatic organ involvement with distant (nonregional) nodal involvement.

Note: The number of lymph node regions involved may be indicated by a subscript (e.g., II_3).
Each stage is subdivided into A or B categories as in Hodgkin's disease (see p. 141).

From AJCC Cancer Staging Handbook. *Philadelphia: Lippincott-Raven, 1998:264.*

OVARIAN CANCER CLASSIFICATION
PRIMARY TUMOR (T)

TNM CATEGORIES		FIGO STAGES	
TX			Primary tumor cannot be assessed
T0			No evidence of primary tumor
T1		I	Tumor limited to ovaries (one or both)
	T1a	IA	Tumor limited to one ovary; capsule intact, no tumor on ovarian surface; no malignant cells in ascites or peritoneal washings*
	T1b	IB	Tumor limited to both ovaries; capsules intact, no tumor on ovarian surface; no malignant cells in ascites or peritoneal washings*
	T1c	IC	Tumor limited to one or both ovaries with any of the following: capsule ruptured, tumor on ovarian surface, malignant cells in ascites or peritoneal washings
T2		II	Tumor involves one or both ovaries with pelvic extension
	T2a	IIA	Extension and/or implants on uterus and/or tube(s); no malignant cells in ascites or peritoneal washings

OVARIAN CANCER CLASSIFICATION *Continued*
PRIMARY TUMOR (T)

TNM CATEGORIES	FIGO STAGES	
T2b	IIB	Extension to other pelvic tissues; no malignant cells in ascites or peritoneal washings
T2c	IIC	Pelvic extension (2a or 2b) with malignant cells in ascites or peritoneal washings
T3 and/or N1	III	Tumor involves one or both ovaries with microscopically confirmed peritoneal metastasis outside the pelvis and/or regional lymph node metastasis
T3a	IIIA	Microscopic peritoneal metastasis beyond pelvis
T3b	IIIB	Macroscopic peritoneal metastasis beyond pelvis 2 cm or less in greatest dimension
T3c and/or N1	IIIC	Peritoneal metastasis beyond pelvis more than 2 cm in greatest dimension and/or regional lymph node metastasis
M1	IV	Distant metastasis (excludes peritoneal metastasis)

REGIONAL LYMPH NODES (N)

NX	Regional lymph nodes cannot be assessed
N0	No regional lymph node metastasis
N1	Regional lymph node metastasis

DISTANT METASTASIS (M)

MX	Distant metastasis cannot be assessed
M0	No distant metastasis
M1	Distant metastasis (excludes peritoneal metastasis)

pTNM PATHOLOGIC CLASSIFICATION
The pT, pN, and pM categories correspond to the T, N, and M categories.

Stage Grouping

Stage IA	T1a	N0	M0
Stage IB	T1b	N0	M0
Stage IC	T1c	N0	M0
Stage IIA	T2a	N0	M0
Stage IIB	T2b	N0	M0
Stage IIC	T2c	N0	M0
Stage IIIA	T3a	N0	M0
Stage IIIB	T3b	N0	M0
Stage IIIC	T3c	N0	M0
	Any T	N1	M0
Stage IV	Any T	Any N	M1

* The presence of nonmalignant ascites is not classified. The presence of ascites does not affect staging unless malignant cells are present.

From AJCC Cancer Staging Handbook. Philadelphia: Lippincott-Raven, 1998:188–189.

PARANASAL SINUSES CANCER CLASSIFICATION

MAXILLARY SINUS
PRIMARY TUMOR (T)

TX	Primary tumor cannot be assessed
T0	No evidence of primary tumor
Tis	Carcinoma in situ
T1	Tumor limited to the antral mucosa with no erosion or destruction of bone
T2	Tumor causing bone erosion or destruction, except for the posterior antral wall, including extension into the hard palate and/or the middle nasal meatus
T3	Tumor invades any of the following: bone of the posterior wall of maxillary sinus, subcutaneous tissues, skin of cheek, floor or medial wall of orbit, infratemporal fossa, pterygoid plates, ethmoid sinuses
T4	Tumor invades orbital contents beyond the floor or medial wall including any of the following: the orbital apex, cribriform plate, base of skull, nasopharynx, sphenoid, frontal sinuses

ETHMOID SINUS
PRIMARY TUMOR (T)

T1	Tumor confined to the ethmoid sinuses with or without bone erosion
T2	Tumor extends into the nasal cavity
T3	Tumor extends to the anterior orbit and/or maxillary sinus
T4	Tumor with intracranial extension, orbital extension including apex, involving sphenoid and/or frontal sinus and/or skin of external nose

REGIONAL LYMPH NODES (N)

NX	Regional lymph nodes cannot be assessed
N0	No regional lymph node metastasis
N1	Metastasis in a single ipsilateral lymph node, 3 cm or less in greatest dimension
N2	Metastasis in a single ipsilateral lymph node, more than 3 cm but not more than 6 cm in greatest dimension, or in multiple ipsilateral lymph nodes, none more than 6 cm in greatest dimension or in bilateral or contralateral lymph nodes, none more than 6 cm in greatest dimension
	N2a Metastasis in a single ipsilateral lymph node more than 3 cm but not more than 6 cm in greatest dimension
	N2b Metastasis in multiple ipsilateral lymph nodes, none more than 6 cm in greatest dimension
	N2c Metastasis in bilateral or contralateral lymph nodes, none more than 6 cm in greatest dimension
N3	Metastasis in a lymph node more than 6 cm in greatest dimension

DISTANT METASTASIS (M)

MX	Distant metastasis cannot be assessed
M0	No distant metastasis
M1	Distant metastasis

PARANASAL SINUSES CANCER CLASSIFICATION *Continued*

Stage Grouping

Stage 0	Tis	N0	M0
Stage I	T1	N0	M0
Stage II	T2	N0	M0
Stage III	T3	N0	M0
	T1	N1	M0
	T2	N1	M0
	T3	N1	M0
Stage IVA	T4	N0	M0
	T4	N1	M0
Stage IVB	Any T	N2	M0
	Any T	N3	M0
Stage IVC	Any T	Any N	M1

From **AJCC Cancer Staging Handbook.** *Philadelphia: Lippincott-Raven, 1998:53–54.*

PENIS CANCER CLASSIFICATION

PRIMARY TUMOR (T)

TX	Primary tumor cannot be assessed
T0	No evidence of primary tumor
Tis	Carcinoma in situ
Ta	Noninvasive verrucous carcinoma
T1	Tumor invades subepithelial connective tissue
T2	Tumor invades corpus spongiosum or cavernosum
T3	Tumor invades urethra or prostate
T4	Tumor invades other adjacent structures

REGIONAL LYMPH NODES (N)

NX	Regional lymph nodes cannot be assessed
N0	No regional lymph node metastasis
N1	Metastasis in a single superficial, inguinal lymph node
N2	Metastasis in multiple or bilateral superficial inguinal lymph nodes
N3	Metastasis in deep inguinal or pelvic lymph node(s) unilateral or bilateral

DISTANT METASTASIS (M)

MX	Distant metastasis cannot be assessed
M0	No distant metastasis
M1	Distant metastasis

Stage Grouping

Stage 0	Tis	N0	M0
	Ta	N0	M0
Stage I	T1	N0	M0
Stage II	T1	N1	M0
	T2	N0	M0
	T2	N1	M0
Stage III	T1	N2	M0
	T2	N2	M0
	T3	N0	M0
	T3	N1	M0
	T3	N2	M0
Stage IV	T4	Any N	M0
	Any T	N3	M0
	Any T	Any N	M1

From AJCC Cancer Staging Handbook. Philadelphia: Lippincott-Raven, 1998:200.

PHARYNGEAL CANCER CLASSIFICATION

PRIMARY TUMOR (T)
TX   Primary tumor cannot be assessed
T0   No evidence of primary tumor
Tis   Carcinoma in situ

Nasopharynx
T1   Tumor confined to the nasopharynx
T2   Tumor extends to soft tissues of oropharynx and/or nasal fossa
         T2a   Without parapharyngeal extension
         T2b   With parapharyngeal extension
T3   Tumor invades bony structures and/or paranasal sinuses
T4   Tumor with intracranial extension and/or involvement of cranial
         nerves, infratemporal fossa, hypopharynx, or orbit

Oropharynx
T1   Tumor 2 cm or less in greatest dimension
T2   Tumor more than 2 cm but not more than 4 cm in greatest
         dimension
T3   Tumor more than 4 cm in greatest dimension
T4   Tumor invades adjacent structures (e.g., pterygoid muscle[s],
         mandible, hard palate, deep muscle of tongue, larynx)

Hypopharynx
T1   Tumor limited to one subsite of hypopharynx and 2 cm or less in
         greatest dimension
T2   Tumor involves more than one subsite of hypopharynx or an
         adjacent site, or measures more than 2 cm but not more than 4 cm
         in greatest diameter without fixation of hemilarynx
T3   Tumor measures more than 4 cm in greatest dimension or with
         fixation of hemilarynx
T4   Tumor invades adjacent structures (e.g., thyroid/cricoid cartilage,
         carotid artery, soft tissues of neck, prevertebral fascia/muscles,
         thyroid and/or esophagus)

REGIONAL LYMPH NODES (N)

Nasopharynx
NX   Regional lymph nodes cannot be assessed
N0   No regional lymph node metastasis
N1   Unilateral metastasis in lymph node(s), 6 cm or less in greatest
         dimension
N2   Bilateral metastasis in lymph node(s), 6 cm or less in greatest
         dimension, above the supraclavicular fossa
N3   Metastasis in a lymph node(s)
         N3a   Greater than 6 cm in dimension
         N3b   Extension to the supraclavicular fossa

Oropharynx and Hypopharynx
NX   Regional lymph nodes cannot be assessed
N0   No regional lymph node metastasis
N1   Metastasis in a single ipsilateral lymph node, 3 cm or less in greatest
         dimension

Table continued on following page

PHARYNGEAL CANCER CLASSIFICATION *Continued*

N2   Metastasis in a single ipsilateral lymph node, more than 3 cm but not more than 6 cm in greatest dimension, or in multiple ipsilateral lymph nodes, none more than 6 cm in greatest dimension, or in bilateral or contralateral lymph nodes, none more than 6 cm in greatest dimension

    N2a   Metastasis in a single ipsilateral lymph node more than 3 cm but not more than 6 cm in greatest dimension

    N2b   Metastasis in multiple ipsilateral lymph nodes, none more than 6 cm in greatest dimension

    N2c   Metastasis in bilateral or contralateral lymph nodes, none more than 6 cm in greatest dimension

N3   Metastasis in a lymph node more than 6 cm in greatest dimension

DISTANT METASTASIS (M)

MX   Distant metastasis cannot be assessed

M0   No distant metastasis

M1   Distant metastasis

Stage Grouping

Nasopharynx

Stage 0	Tis	N0	M0
Stage I	T1	N0	M0
Stage IIA	T2a	N0	M0
Stage IIB	T1	N1	M0
	T2	N1	M0
	T2a	N1	M0
	T2b	N0	M0
	T2b	N1	M0
Stage III	T1	N2	M0
	T2a	N2	M0
	T2b	N2	M0
	T3	N0	M0
	T3	N1	M0
	T3	N2	M0
Stage IVA	T4	N0	M0
	T4	N1	M0
	T4	N2	M0
Stage IVB	Any T	N3	M0
Stage IVC	Any T	Any N	M1

Oropharynx and Hypopharynx

Stage 0	Tis	N0	M0
Stage I	T1	N0	M0
Stage II	T2	N0	M0
Stage III	T3	N0	M0
	T1	N1	M0
	T2	N1	M0
	T3	N1	M0

PHARYNGEAL CANCER CLASSIFICATION *Continued*

Stage IVA	T4	N0	M0
	T4	N1	M0
	Any T	N2	M0
Stage IVB	Any T	N3	M0
Stage IVC	Any T	Any N	M1

*From **AJCC Cancer Staging Handbook**. Philadelphia: Lippincott-Raven, 1998:38–40.*

PLEURAL MESOTHELIOMA CLASSIFICATION

PRIMARY TUMOR (T)

TX	Primary tumor cannot be assessed
T0	No evidence of primary tumor
T1	Tumor limited to ipsilateral parietal and/or visceral pleura
T2	Tumor invades any of the following: ipsilateral lung, endothoracic fascia, diaphragm, pericardium
T3	Tumor invades any of the following: ipsilateral chest wall muscle, ribs, mediastinal organs or tissues
T4	Tumor directly extends to any of the following: contralateral pleura, lung, peritoneum, intraabdominal organs, or cervical tissues

REGIONAL LYMPH NODES (N)

NX	Regional lymph nodes cannot be assessed
N0	No regional lymph node metastasis
N1	Metastasis in ipsilateral peribronchial and/or ipsilateral hilar lymph nodes, including direct extension
N2	Metastasis in ipsilateral mediastinal and/or subcarinal lymph node(s)
N3	Metastasis in contralateral mediastinal, contralateral hilar, ipsilateral or contralateral scalene, or supraclavicular lymph node(s)

DISTANT METASTASIS (M)

MX	Distant metastasis cannot be assessed
M0	No evidence of distant metastasis
M1	Distant metastasis

Stage Grouping

Stage I	T1	N0	M0
	T2	N0	M0
Stage II	T1	N1	M0
	T2	N1	M0
Stage III	T1	N2	M0
	T2	N2	M0
	T3	N0	M0
	T3	N1	M0
	T3	N2	M0
Stage IV	Any T	N3	M0
	T4	Any N	M0
	Any T	Any N	M1

*From **AJCC Cancer Staging Handbook**. Philadelphia: Lippincott-Raven, 1998:129–130.*

PROSTATE CANCER CLASSIFICATION

PRIMARY TUMOR

Clinical (T)

TX   Primary tumor cannot be assessed
T0   No evidence of primary tumor
T1   Clinically inapparent tumor not palpable nor visible by imaging
      T1a   Tumor incidental histologic finding in 5% or less of tissue resected
      T1b   Tumor incidental histologic finding in more than 5% of tissue resected
      T1c   Tumor identified by needle biopsy (e.g., because of elevated prostate-specific antigen)
T2   Tumor confined within prostate*
      T2a   Tumor involves one lobe
      T2b   Tumor involves both lobes
T3   Tumor extends through the prostate capsule†
      T3a   Extracapsular extension (unilateral or bilateral)
      T3b   Tumor invades seminal vesicle(s)
T4   Tumor is fixed or invades adjacent structures other than seminal vesicles: bladder neck, external sphincter, rectum, levator muscles, and/or pelvic wall

Pathologic (pT)

pT2‡   Organ confined
      pT2a   Unilateral
      pT2b   Bilateral
pT3   Extraprostatic extension
      pT3a   Extraprostatic extension
      pT3b   Seminal vesicle invasion
pT4   Invasion of bladder, rectum

REGIONAL LYMPH NODES (N)

NX   Regional lymph nodes cannot be assessed
N0   No regional lymph node metastasis
N1   Metastasis in regional lymph node or nodes

DISTANT METASTASIS§ (M)

MX   Distant metastasis cannot be assessed
M0   No distant metastasis
M1   Distant metastasis
      M1a   Nonregional lymph node(s)
      M1b   Bone(s)
      M1c   Other site(s)

HISTOPATHOLOGIC GRADE (G)

GX   Grade cannot be assessed
G1   Well differentiated (slight anaplasia)
G2   Moderately differentiated (moderate anaplasia)
G3-4   Poorly differentiated or undifferentiated (marked anaplasia)

PROSTATE CANCER CLASSIFICATION *Continued*

Stage Grouping

Stage I	T1a	N0	M0	G1
Stage II	T1a	N0	M0	G2, 3-4
	T1b	N0	M0	Any G
	T1c	N0	M0	Any G
	T1	N0	M0	Any G
	T2	N0	M0	Any G
Stage III	T3	N0	M0	Any G
Stage IV	T4	N0	M0	Any G
	Any T	N1	M0	Any G
	Any T	Any N	M1	Any G

* Tumor found in one or both lobes by needle biopsy, but not palpable or reliably visible by imaging, is classified as T1c.

† Invasion into the prostatic apex or into (but not beyond) the prostatic capsule is not classified as T3, but as T2.

‡ There is no pathologic T1 classification.

§ When more than one site of metastasis is present, the most advanced category is used. pM1c is most advanced.

From AJCC Cancer Staging Handbook. *Philadelphia: Lippincott-Raven, 1998:205–206.*

RENAL PELVIS AND URETER CANCER CLASSIFICATION

PRIMARY TUMOR (T)

TX	Primary tumor cannot be assessed
T0	No evidence of primary tumor
Ta	Papillary noninvasive carcinoma
Tis	Carcinoma in situ
T1	Tumor invades subepithelial connective tissue
T2	Tumor invades the muscularis
T3	For renal pelvis only: tumor invades beyond muscularis into peripelvic fat or the renal parenchyma
T3	For ureter only: tumor invades beyond muscularis into periureteric fat
T4	Tumor invades adjacent organs, or through the kidney into the perinephric fat

REGIONAL LYMPH NODES (N)*

NX	Regional lymph nodes cannot be assessed
N0	No regional lymph node metastasis
N1	Metastasis in a single lymph node, 2 cm or less in greatest dimension
N2	Metastasis in a single lymph node, more than 2 cm but not more than 5 cm in greatest dimension; or multiple lymph nodes, none more than 5 cm in greatest dimension
N3	Metastasis in a lymph node more than 5 cm in greatest dimension

DISTANT METASTASIS (M)

MX	Distant metastasis cannot be assessed
M0	No distant metastasis
M1	Distant metastasis

Stage Grouping

Stage 0a	Ta	N0	M0
Stage 0is	Tis	N0	M0
Stage I	T1	N0	M0
Stage II	T2	N0	M0
Stage III	T3	N0	M0
Stage IV	T4	N0	M0
	Any T	N1	M0
	Any T	N2	M0
	Any T	N3	M0
	Any T	Any N	M1

* Laterality does not affect the N classification.

*From **AJCC Cancer Staging Handbook**. Philadelphia: Lippincott-Raven, 1998:220–221.*

RETINOBLASTOMA CLASSIFICATION

PRIMARY TUMOR (T)

TX	Primary tumor cannot be assessed
T0	No evidence of primary tumor
T1	Tumor(s) limited to 25% or less of the retina
T2	Tumor(s) involve(s) more than 25% but not more than 50% of the retina
T3	Tumor(s) involve(s) more than 50% of the retina and/or invade(s) beyond the retina but remain(s) intraocular

    T3a   Tumor(s) involve(s) more than 50% of the retina and/or tumor cells in the vitreous

    T3b   Tumor(s) involve(s) optic disc

    T3c   Tumor(s) involve(s) anterior chamber and/or uvea

T4	Tumor with extraocular invasion

    T4a   Tumor invades retrobulbar optic nerve

    T4b   Extraocular extension other than invasion of optic nerve

REGIONAL LYMPH NODES (N)

NX	Regional lymph nodes cannot be assessed
N0	No regional lymph node metastasis
N1	Regional lymph node metastasis

DISTANT METASTASIS (M)

MX	Distant metastasis cannot be assessed
M0	No distant metastasis
M1	Distant metastasis

PATHOLOGIC CLASSIFICATION (pTNM)

Primary Tumor (T)

pTX	Primary tumor cannot be assessed
pT0	No evidence of primary tumor
pT1	Tumor(s) limited to 25% or less of the retina
pT2	Tumor(s) involve(s) more than 25% but not more than 50% of the retina
pT3	Tumor(s) involve(s) more than 50% of the retina and/or invade(s) beyond the retina but remain(s) intraocular

    pT3a   Tumor(s) involve(s) more than 50% of the retina and/or tumor cells in the vitreous

    pT3b   Tumor(s) invades optic nerve as far as the lamina cribrosa

    pT3c   Tumor in anterior chamber and/or invasion with thickening of the uvea and/or intrascleral invasion

pT4	Tumor with extraocular invasion

    pT4a   Intraneural tumor beyond the lamina cribrosa but not at the line of resection

    pT4b   Tumor at the line of resection or other extraocular extension

Regional Lymph Nodes (pN)

pNX	Regional lymph nodes cannot be assessed
pN0	No regional lymph node metastasis
pN1	Regional lymph node metastasis

Table continued on following page

RETINOBLASTOMA CLASSIFICATION *Continued*

Distant Metastasis (pM)

pMX   Distant metastasis cannot be assessed
pM0   No distant metastasis
pM1   Distant metastasis

Stage Grouping

In cases of bilateral disease the more affected eye is used for the stage grouping.

Stage IA	T1	N0	M0
Stage IB	T2	N0	M0
Stage IIA	T3a	N0	M0
Stage IIB	T3b	N0	M0
Stage IIC	T3c	N0	M0
Stage IIIA	T4a	N0	M0
Stage IIIB	T4b	N0	M0
Stage IV	Any T	N1	M0
	Any T	Any N	M1

Note: Pathologic stage grouping corresponds to the clinical stage grouping.

From AJCC Cancer Staging Handbook. *Philadelphia: Lippincott-Raven, 1998:247–249.*

SARCOMA OF THE ORBIT CLASSIFICATION

PRIMARY TUMOR (T)

TX   Primary tumor cannot be assessed
T0   No evidence of primary tumor
T1   Tumor 15 mm or less in greatest dimension
T2   Tumor more than 15 mm in greatest dimension
T3   Tumor of any size with diffuse invasion of orbital tissues and/or bony walls
T4   Tumor invades beyond the orbit to adjacent sinuses and/or to cranium

REGIONAL LYMPH NODES (N)

NX   Regional lymph nodes cannot be assessed
N0   No regional lymph node metastasis
N1   Regional lymph node metastasis

DISTANT METASTASIS (M)

MX   Distant metastasis cannot be assessed
M0   No distant metastasis
M1   Distant metastasis

Stage Grouping

No stage grouping presently is recommended.

From AJCC Cancer Staging Handbook. *Philadelphia: Lippincott-Raven, 1998:253–254.*

SMALL INTESTINE CANCER CLASSIFICATION

PRIMARY TUMOR (T)

TX	Primary tumor cannot be assessed
T0	No evidence of primary tumor
Tis	Carcinoma in situ
T1	Tumor invades lamina propria or submucosa
T2	Tumor invades muscularis propria
T3	Tumor invades through the muscularis propria into the subserosa or into the nonperitonealized perimuscular tissue (mesentery or retroperitoneum) with extension 2 cm or less*
T4	Tumor perforates the visceral peritoneum, or directly invades other organs or structures (includes other loops of small intestine, mesentery, or retroperitoneum more than 2 cm, and abdominal wall by way of serosa; for duodenum only, invasion of pancreas)

REGIONAL LYMPH NODES (N)

NX	Regional lymph nodes cannot be assessed
N0	No regional lymph node metastasis
N1	Regional lymph node metastasis

DISTANT METASTASIS (M)

MX	Distant metastasis cannot be assessed
M0	No distant metastasis
M1	Distant metastasis

Stage Grouping

Stage 0	Tis	N0	M0
Stage I	T1	N0	M0
	T2	N0	M0
Stage II	T3	N0	M0
	T4	N0	M0
Stage III	Any T	N1	M0
Stage IV	Any T	Any N	M1

* The nonperitonealized perimuscular tissue is, for jejunum and ileum, part of the mesentery and, for duodenum in areas where serosa is lacking, part of the retroperitoneum.

*From **AJCC Cancer Staging Handbook**. Philadelphia: Lippincott-Raven, 1998:78–79.*

SOFT TISSUE SARCOMA CLASSIFICATION

PRIMARY TUMOR (P)

TX   Primary tumor cannot be assessed
T0   No evidence of primary tumor
T1   Tumor 5 cm or less in greatest dimension
          T1a   Superficial tumor
          T1b   Deep tumor
T2   Tumor more than 5 cm in greatest dimension
          T2a   Superficial tumor
          T2b   Deep tumor

REGIONAL LYMPH NODES (N)

NX   Regional lymph nodes cannot be assessed
N0   No regional lymph node metastasis
N1   Regional lymph node metastasis

DISTANT METASTASIS (M)

MX   Distant metastasis cannot be found
M0   No distant metastasis
M1   Distant metastasis

HISTOPATHOLOGIC GRADE (G)

GX   Grade cannot be assessed
G1   Well differentiated
G2   Moderately differentiated
G3   Poorly differentiated
G4   Undifferentiated

Stage Grouping

Stage I				
A (Low grade, small, superficial and deep)	G1-2	T1a-1b	N0	M0
B (Low grade, large, superficial)	G1-2	T2a	N0	M0
Stage II				
A (Low grade, large, deep)	G1-2,	T2b	N0	M0
B (High grade, small, superficial, deep)	G3-4,	T1a-1b	N0	M0
C (High grade, large, superficial)	G3-4,	T2a	N0	M0
Stage III (High grade, large, deep)	G3-4,	T2b	N0	M0
Stage IV (Any metastasis)	Any G	Any T	N0	M1
	Any G	Any T	N1	M0

From **AJCC Cancer Staging Handbook.** *Philadelphia: Lippincott-Raven, 1998:143–144.*

STOMACH CANCER CLASSIFICATION

PRIMARY TUMOR (T)

TX   Primary tumor cannot be assessed
T0   No evidence of primary tumor
Tis   Carcinoma in situ: intra-epithelial tumor without invasion of the lamina propria

STOMACH CANCER CLASSIFICATION *Continued*

T1	Tumor invades lamina propria or submucosa
T2	Tumor invades muscularis propria or subserosa*
T3	Tumor penetrates serosa (visceral peritoneum) without invasion of adjacent structures†‡
T4	Tumor invades adjacent structures†‡

REGIONAL LYMPH NODES (N)

NX	Regional lymph node(s) cannot be assessed
N0	No regional lymph node metastasis
N1	Metastasis in 1 to 6 regional lymph nodes
N2	Metastasis in 7 to 15 regional lymph nodes
N3	Metastasis in more than 15 regional lymph nodes

DISTANT METASTASIS (M)

MX	Distant metastasis cannot be assessed
M0	No distant metastasis
M1	Distant metastasis

Stage Grouping

Stage 0	Tis	N0	M0
Stage IA	T1	N0	M0
Stage IB	T1	N1	M0
	T2	N0	M0
Stage II	T1	N2	M0
	T2	N1	M0
	T3	N0	M0
Stage IIIA	T2	N2	M0
	T3	N1	M0
	T4	N0	M0
Stage IIIB	T3	N2	M0
Stage IV	T4	N1	M0
	T1	N3	M0
	T2	N3	M0
	T3	N3	M0
	T4	N2	M0
	T4	N3	M0
	Any T	Any N	M1

* A tumor may penetrate the muscularis propria with extension into the gastrocolic or gastrophepatic ligaments, or into the greater or lesser omentum without perforation of the visceral peritoneum covering these structures. In this case, the tumor is classified T2. If there is perforation of the visceral peritoneum covering the gastric ligaments or the omentum, the tumor should be classified T3.

† The adjacent structures of the stomach include the spleen, transverse colon, liver, diaphragm, pancreas, abdominal wall, adrenal gland, kidney, small intestine, and retroperitoneum.

‡ Intramural extension to the duodenum or esophagus is classified by the depth of greatest invasion in any of these sites, including stomach.

*From **AJCC Cancer Staging Handbook**. Philadelphia: Lippincott-Raven, 1998:73–74.*

TESTIS CANCER CLASSIFICATION

PRIMARY TUMOR (pT)

The extent of primary tumor is classified after radical orchiectomy.

pTX   Primary tumor cannot be assessed (if no radical orchiectomy has been performed; TX is used)

pT0   No evidence of primary tumor (e.g., histologic scar in testis)

pTis   Intratubular germ cell neoplasia (carcinoma in situ)

pT1   Tumor limited to the testis and epididymis without vascular/lymphatic invasion; tumor may invade into the tunica albuginea but not the tunica vaginalis

pT2   Tumor limited to the testis and epididymis with vascular/lymphatic involvement of the tunica vaginalis

pT3   Tumor invades the spermatic cord with or without vascular/lymphatic invasion

pT4   Tumor invades the scrotum with or without vascular/lymphatic invasion

REGIONAL LYMPH NODES (N)

Clinical

NX   Regional lymph nodes cannot be assessed

N0   No regional lymph node metastasis

N1   Metastasis with a lymph node mass 2 cm or less in greatest dimension; or multiple lymph nodes, none more than 2 cm in greatest dimension

N2   Metastasis with a lymph node mass, more than 2 cm but not more than 5 cm in greatest dimension; or multiple lymph nodes, any one mass greater than 2 cm but not more than 5 cm in greatest dimension

N3   Metastasis with a lymph node mass more than 5 cm in greatest dimension

Pathologic (pN)

pNX   Regional lymph nodes cannot be assessed

pN0   No regional lymph node metastasis

pN1   Metastasis with a lymph node mass, 2 cm or less in greatest dimension and less than or equal to 5 nodes positive, none more than 2 cm in greatest dimension

pN2   Metastasis with a lymph node mass, more than 2 cm but not more than 5 cm in greatest dimension; or more than 5 nodes positive, none more than 5 cm; or evidence of extranodal extension of tumor

pN3   Metastasis with a lymph node mass more than 5 cm in greatest dimension

DISTANT METASTASIS (M)

MX   Distant metastasis cannot be assessed

M0   No distant metastasis

M1   Distant metastasis

      M1a   Nonregional nodal or pulmonary metastasis

      M1b   Distant metastasis other than to nonregional lymph nodes and lungs

TESTIS CANCER CLASSIFICATION *Continued*

SERUM TUMOR MARKERS (S)

SX	Marker studies not available or not performed
S0	Marker study levels within normal limits
S1	LDH $< 1.5 \times$ N AND
hCG	(mIu/mL) < 5000 AND
AFP	(ng/mL) < 1000
S2	LDH $1.5-10 \times$ N OR
hCG	(mIu/mL) 5000–50,000 OR
AFP	(ng/mL) 1000–10,000
S3	LDH $> 10 \times$ N OR
hCG	(mIu/mL) $> 50,000$ OR
AFP	(ng/mL) $> 10,000$
N	Indicates the upper limit of normal for the LDH assay

Stage Grouping

Stage 0	pTis	N0	M0	S0
Stage I	pT1-4	N0	M0	SX
Stage IA	pT1	N0	M0	S0
Stage IB	pT2	N0	M0	S0
	pT3	N0	M0	S0
	pT4	N0	M0	S0
Stage IS	Any pT/Tx	N0	M0	S1-3
Stage II	Any pT/Tx	N1-3	M0	SX
Stage IIA	Any pT/Tx	N1	M0	S0
	Any pT/Tx	N1	M0	S1
Stage IIB	Any pT/Tx	N2	M0	S0
	Any pT/Tx	N2	M0	S1
Stage IIC	Any pT/Tx	N3	M0	S0
	Any pT/Tx	N3	M0	S1
Stage III	Any pT/Tx	Any N	M1	SX
Stage IIIA	Any pT/Tx	Any N	M1a	S0
	Any pT/Tx	Any N	M1a	S1
Stage IIIB	Any pT/Tx	N1-3	M0	S2
	Any pT/Tx	Any N	M1a	S2
Stage IIIC	Any pT/Tx	N1-3	M0	S3
	Any pT/Tx	Any N	M1a	S3
	Any pT/Tx	Any N	M1b	Any S

AFP, alpha-fetoprotein; hCG, human chorionic gonadotropin; LDH, lactate dehydrogenase.

*From **AJCC Cancer Staging Handbook**. Philadelphia: Lippincott-Raven, 1998:210–212.*

URINARY BLADDER CANCER CLASSIFICATION

PRIMARY TUMOR (T)

TX	Primary tumor cannot be assessed
T0	No evidence of primary tumor
Ta	Noninvasive papillary carcinoma
Tis	Carcinoma in situ: "flat tumor"
T1	Tumor invades subepithelial connective tissue
T2	Tumor invades muscle
	T2a Tumor invades superficial muscle (inner half)
	T2b Tumor invades deep muscle (outer half)
T3	Tumor invades perivesical tissue
	T3a Microscopically
	T3b Macroscopically (extravesical mass)
T4	Tumor invades any of the following: prostate, uterus, vagina, pelvic wall, abdominal wall
	T4a Tumor invades prostate, uterus, vagina
	T4b Tumor invades pelvic wall, abdominal wall

REGIONAL LYMPH NODES (N)

Regional lymph nodes are those within the true pelvis; all others are distant lymph nodes.

NX	Regional lymph nodes cannot be assessed
N0	No regional lymph node metastasis
N1	Metastasis in a single lymph node, 2 cm or less in greatest dimension
N2	Metastasis in a single lymph node, more than 2 cm but not more than 5 cm in greatest dimension; or multiple lymph nodes, none more than 5 cm in greatest dimension
N3	Metastasis in a lymph node more than 5 cm in greatest dimension

DISTANT METASTASIS (M)

MX	Distant metastasis cannot be assessed
M0	No distant metastasis
M1	Distant metastasis

Stage Grouping

Stage 0a	Ta	N0	M0
Stage 0is	Tis	N0	M0
Stage I	T1	N0	M0
Stage II	T2a	N0	M0
	T2b	N0	M0
Stage III	T3a	N0	M0
	T3b	N0	M0
	T4a	N0	M0
Stage IV	T4b	N0	M0
	Any T	N1	M0
	Any T	N2	M0
	Any T	N3	M0
	Any T	Any N	M1

From AJCC Cancer Staging Handbook. Philadelphia: Lippincott-Raven, 1998:224–225.

VAGINAL CANCER CLASSIFICATION

PRIMARY TUMOR (T)

TNM CATEGORIES	FIGO STAGES	
TX		Primary tumor cannot be assessed
T0		No evidence of primary tumor
Tis	0	Carcinoma in situ
T1	I	Tumor confined to vagina
T2	II	Tumor invades paravaginal tissues but not to pelvic wall
T3	III	Tumor extends to pelvic wall
T4*	IVA	Tumor invades mucosa of the bladder or rectum and/or extends beyond the true pelvis (bullous edema is not sufficient evidence to classify a tumor as T4)
M1	IVB	Distant metastasis

REGIONAL LYMPH NODES (N)

NX	Regional lymph nodes cannot be assessed
N0	No regional lymph node metastasis
N1	Pelvic or inguinal lymph node metastasis

DISTANT METASTASIS (M)

MX	Distant metastasis cannot be assessed
M0	No distant metastasis
M1	Distant metastasis

pTNM PATHOLOGIC CLASSIFICATION

The pT, pN, and pM categories correspond to the T, N, and M categories.

Stage Grouping

Stage 0	Tis	N0	M0
Stage I	T1	N0	M0
Stage II	T2	N0	M0
Stage III	T1	N1	M0
	T2	N1	M0
	T3	N0	M0
	T3	N1	M0
Stage IVA	T4	Any N	M0
Stage IVB	Any T	Any N	M1

* If the bladder mucosa is not involved, the tumor is Stage III.

From **AJCC Cancer Staging Handbook**. *Philadelphia: Lippincott-Raven, 1998:176–177.*

VULVA CANCER CLASSIFICATION

PRIMARY TUMOR (T)

TX   Primary tumor cannot be assessed
T0   No evidence of primary tumor
Tis   Carcinoma in situ (preinvasive carcinoma)
T1   Tumor confined to the vulva or vulva and perineum, 2 cm or less in greatest dimension

    T1a   Tumor confined to the vulva or vulva and perineum, 2 cm or less in greatest dimension, and with stromal invasion no greater than 1mm*

    T1b   Tumor confined to the vulva or vulva and perineum, 2 cm or less in greatest dimension, and with stromal invasion greater than 1 mm*

T2   Tumor confined to the vulva or vulva and perineum, more than 2 cm in greatest dimension
T3   Tumor of any size with adjacent spread to the lower urethra and/or vagina or anus
T4   Tumor invades any of the following: upper urethral mucosa, bladder mucosa, rectal mucosa, or is fixed to the pubic bone

REGIONAL LYMPH NODES (N)

NX   Regional lymph nodes cannot be assessed
N0   No regional lymph node metastasis
N1   Unilateral regional lymph node metastasis
N2   Bilateral regional lymph node metastasis

DISTANT METASTASIS (M)

MX   Distant metastasis cannot be assessed
M0   No distant metastasis
M1   Distant metastasis (including pelvic lymph node metastasis)

Stage Grouping

Stage 0	Tis	N0	M0
Stage IA	T1a	N0	M0
Stage IB	T1b	N0	M0
Stage II	T2	N0	M0
Stage III	T1	N1	M0
	T2	N1	M0
	T3	N0	M0
	T3	N1	M0
Stage IVA	T1	N2	M0
	T2	N2	M0
	T3	N2	M0
	T4	Any N	M0
Stage IVB	Any T	Any N	M1

* The depth of invasion is defined as the measurement of the tumor from the epithelial-stromal junction of the adjacent most superficial dermal papilla to the deepest point of invasion.

From AJCC Cancer Staging Handbook. *Philadelphia: Lippincott-Raven, 1998:172–173.*

STAGING OF MESOTHELIOMA
▷ (Proposed by Chahinian)

STAGE	DESCRIPTION
I	T1, N0, M0
II	T1-2, N1, M0
	T2, N0, M0
III	T3, any N, M0
IV	T4, any N, M0, any M1

T = PRIMARY TUMOR
  T1 = Limited to ipsilateral pleura only
  T2 = Superficial local invasion
  T3 = Deep local invasion
  T4 = Extensive direct invasion

N = LYMPH NODES
  N0 = No positive lymph node
  N1 = Positive ipsilateral hilar node
  N2 = Positive mediastinal nodes
  N3 = Positive contralateral hilar nodes

M = METASTASIS
  M0 = No metastasis
  M1 = Blood-borne or lymphatic metastasis

From Chahinian AP: Therapeutic modalities in malignant pleural mesothelioma. In Chretien J, Hirsch A (eds): Diseases of the Pleura. New York: Masson, 1983.

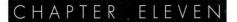

CHAPTER ELEVEN

Urology

GRADING OF ENURESIS

TYPE	CYSTOMETRIC FINDINGS	ELECTROENCEPHALOGRAM FINDINGS
I	Stable bladder	Positive response during an enuretic episode
IIa	Stable bladder	No response during an enuretic episode
IIb	Unstable bladder	No response during an enuretic episode

From Watanabe H, Azuma Y: A proposal for a classification system of enuresis based on overnight simultaneous monitoring of EEG and cystometry. Sleep 1989; 12:257–264.

TYPES OF HYPEROXALURIA

TYPE	DESCRIPTION
I	Increased oxalate production (primary hyperoxaluria, increased hepatic conversion)
II	Increased oxalate absorption
III	Idiopathic calcium oxalate stone disease

From Walsh PC, Retik AB, Vaughan ED, et al. (eds): Campbell's Urology, 7th ed. Philadelphia: W.B. Saunders, 1998:2681.

UTERINE PROLAPSE GRADING

GRADE	CLINICAL FINDING
1	Descent of cervix toward introitus with straining
2	Descent of cervix to the level of the introitus with straining
3	Cervix outside introitus with straining
4	Cervix outside introitus at rest

From Walsh PC, Retik AB, Vaughan ED, et al. (eds): Campbell's Urology, 7th ed. Philadelphia: W.B. Saunders, 1998:1075.

AMERICAN UROLOGICAL ASSOCIATION (AUA) SYMPTOM INDEX FOR BENIGN PROSTATIC HYPERPLASIA

QUESTION	NOT AT ALL	LESS THAN 1 TIME IN 5	LESS THAN HALF THE TIME	HALF THE TIME	MORE THAN HALF THE TIME	ALMOST ALWAYS
During the last month, how often have you had a sensation of not emptying your bladder completely after you finished urinating?	0	1	2	3	4	5
During the last month, how often have you had to urinate again less than 2 hours after you finished urinating?	0	1	2	3	4	5
During the last month, how often have you found you stopped and started again several times when you urinated?	0	1	2	3	4	5

During the last month, how often have you found it difficult to postpone urination?	0	1	2	3	4	5
During the last month, how often have you had a weak urinary system?	0	1	2	3	4	5
During the last month, how often have you had to push or strain to begin urination?	0	1	2	3	4	5
During the last month, how many times did you most typically get up to urinate from the time you went to bed at night until the time you got up in the morning?	0	1	2	3	4	5

AUA symptom score = sum of questions 1 to 7.
The index is very sensitive to change and helpful in quantitating symptoms before and after surgery.

From Barry MJ, Fowler FJ Jr., O'Leary MP, et al.: The AUA symptom index for BPH. J Urol 1992; 148:1555.

DEVINE AND HORTON CLASSIFICATION OF CONGENITAL PENILE CURVATURE

CLASS	DESCRIPTION
I	Epithelial urethra beneath the skin. Dysgenic tissue beneath it represents undeveloped corpus spongiosum, Buck's fascia, and dartos fascia
II	Normal urethra and spongiosum but abnormal Buck's and dartos fascia
III	Abnormal dartos fascia only
IV	Normal urethra and fascial layers with abnormal corpocavernosal development
V	Congenital short urethra

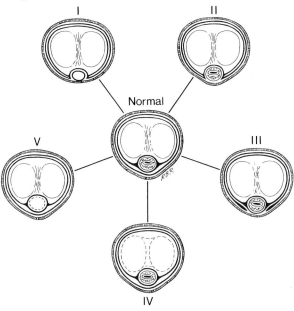

From Devine CJ, Horton CE: Bent penis. Semin Urol 1987; 5:252.

PELVIC MUSCLE RATING SCALE (LEVATOR FUNCTION)

	1	2	3	4
Pressure	None	Weak	Moderate	Strong
Duration	None	<1 sec	1–5 sec	>5 sec
Displacement	None	Slight anterior	Whole anterior	Gripped

This rating scale assesses levator function during routine bimanual pelvic examination.

From Walsh PC, Retik AB, Vaughan ED, et al. (eds): Campbell's Urology, 7th ed. Philadelphia: W.B. Saunders, 1998:1032.

RECTOCELE GRADING

GRADE	CLINICAL FINDING
Low	Separation of the levator ani and bulbocavernosus from the perineal body
Mid	Bulging of rectum into the vagina above the levator hiatus; separation of pararectal and prerectal fascia
High	Bulging of rectum into the upper vaginal vault, frequently associated with an enterocele

From Walsh PC, Retik AB, Vaughan ED, et al. (eds): Campbell's Urology, 7th ed. Philadelphia: W.B. Saunders, 1998:1075.

CYSTOCELE GRADING

GRADE	CLINICAL FINDING
1	Descent of bladder base toward introitus with straining
2	Descent of bladder base to the level of the introitus with straining
3	Descent of bladder base outside the introitus with straining
4	Bladder base outside introitus at rest

A cystocele is the descent of the bladder base below the inferior ramus of the pubic symphysis.

From Walsh PC, Retik AB, Vaughan ED, et al. (eds): Campbell's Urology, 7th ed. Philadelphia: W.B. Saunders, 1998:1075.

INCONTINENCE GRADING SYSTEM (SUBJECTIVE)

GRADE	SUBJECTIVE FINDING
0	Continent
I	Patient loses urine with a sudden increase in abdominal pressure but not supine
II	Patient loses urine with physical stress (walking, changing from a reclining to a standing position, sitting up in bed)
III	Patient with total incontinence; urine loss unrelated to physical activity and/or position

In this system, an improvement in continence is noted when the patient reports a decrease in the grade of incontinence.

Adapted from Walsh PC, Retik AB, Vaughan ED, et al. (eds): Campbell's Urology, 7th ed. Philadelphia: W.B. Saunders, 1998:1023.

CATEGORIZATION OF PRUNE-BELLY SYNDROME

CATEGORY	FINDINGS
I	Oligohydramnios, pulmonary hypoplasia, or pneumothorax; may have urethral obstruction or patent urachus and club foot
II	Typical external features and uropathy of the full-blown syndrome but no immediate problem with survival; may have mild or unilateral renal dysplasia; may or may not develop urosepsis or gradual azotemia
III	External features may be mild or incomplete; uropathy is less severe; renal function is stable

From Walsh PC, Retik AB, Vaughan ED, et al. (eds): Campbell's Urology, 7th ed. Philadelphia: W.B. Saunders, 1998:1923.

CLASSIFICATION OF POSTERIOR URETHRAL VALVES

TYPE	ANATOMIC FINDING
I	An obstructing membrane that radiates in a distal direction from the posterior edge of the verumontanum toward the membranous urethra, inserting anteriorly near the proximal margin of the membranous urethra
II	Hypertrophy of the strip of superficial muscle that runs from the ureteral orifice to the verumontanum
III	Incomplete dissolution of the urogenital membrane: the obstructing membranes are distal to the verumontanum at the level of the membranous urethra

Type I valves make up 95% of the lesions, with Type III making up the rest. True Type II valves do not exist. The presentation of Type I and III valves is the same, as are the treatments.

From Walsh PC, Retik AB, Vaughan ED, et al. (eds): Campbell's Urology, 7th ed. Philadelphia: W.B. Saunders, 1998: 2069–2070.

ANATOMIC CLASSIFICATION OF URINARY STRESS INCONTINENCE

TYPE	DESCRIPTION
0	Patient complains of stress incontinence, but no urinary leakage is demonstrated during the clinical and urodynamic testing. Vesical neck and proximal urethra are closed at rest and situated at or above the lower end of the symphysis pubis. During stress, the vesical neck and proximal urethra descend and open.
I	The vesical neck is closed at rest and situated above the inferior margin of the symphysis. During stress, the vesical neck and proximal urethra open and descend less than 2 cm, and urinary incontinence is apparent during periods of increased abdominal pressure. There is a small or no cystocele.
IIA	The vesical neck is closed at rest and situated above the inferior margin of the symphysis pubis. During stress, the neck and proximal urethra open, and there is rotational descent characteristic of a cystourethrocele. Incontinence is apparent during periods of increased abdominal pressure.
IIB	The vesical neck is closed at rest and situated at or below the inferior margin of the symphysis. During stress, there may or may not be further descent, but the proximal urethra opens and incontinence ensues.
III	The vesical neck and proximal urethra are open at rest in the absence of a detrusor contraction. The proximal urethra no longer functions as a sphincter. There is obvious leakage.

From Walsh PC, Retik AB, Vaughan ED, et al. (eds): Campbell's Urology, 7th ed. Philadelphia: W.B. Saunders, 1998:1014–1016.

INTERNATIONAL CLASSIFICATION OF VESICOURETERAL REFLUX

GRADE	RADIOGRAPHIC FINDING ON VOIDING CYSTOURETHROGRAPHY (VCUG)
I	Contrast into the nondilated ureter
II	Contrast into the pelvis and calyces without dilation
III	Mild to moderate dilation of the ureter, renal pelvis, and calyces with minimal blunting of the fornices
IV	Moderate ureteral tortuosity and dilation of the pelvis and calyces
V	Gross dilation of the ureter, pelvis, and calyces, loss of papillary impressions, and ureteral tortuosity

This grading system categorizes reflux based on the radiographic findings observed during voiding cystourethrography.

From Walsh PC, Retik AB, Vaughan ED, et al. (eds): Campbell's Urology, 7th ed. Philadelphia: W.B. Saunders, 1998:1865.

TANNER STAGING OF FEMALE PUBIC HAIR DEVELOPMENT

STAGE	DESCRIPTION
1	No pubic hair; preadolescent
2	Sparse, lightly pigmented, straight along medial border of labia
3	Darker, beginning to curl, increased amount
4	Coarse, curly, abundant amount but less than adult
5	Adult female triangle, spread to medial surface of thighs

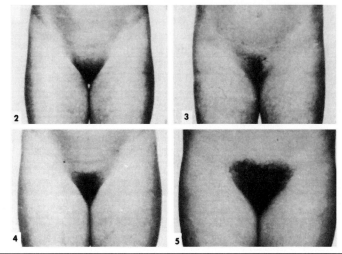

From Seidel HM, Ball JW, Dains JE, Benedict GW: Mosby's Guide to Physical Examination. St. Louis: Mosby, 1987:78.

HISTOLOGIC GRADING OF SCHISTOSOMAL URINARY BLADDER DISEASE

GRADE	CRITERIA
1	Occasional eggs in lamina propria
2	Lamina propria filled with eggs, no involvement of detrusor muscle
3	Lamina propria filled with eggs, involvement of superficial third of detrusor muscle
4	Lamina propria filled with eggs, involvement of external two thirds of detrusor muscle

From Edington GM, Von Lichtenberg F, et al.: Pathologic effects of schistosomiasis in Ibidan, western state of Nigeria. Am J Trop Med Hyg 1970; 19:982.

TANNER STAGING OF MALE GENITAL DEVELOPMENT

STAGE	DESCRIPTION
1	Penis, testes, and scrotum are preadolescent
2	Enlargement of scrotum and testes, texture alteration; scrotal sac reddens; penis usually does not enlarge
3	Further growth of testes and scrotum; penis enlarges and becomes longer
4	Continued growth of testes and scrotum; scrotum becomes darker; penis becomes longer; glans and breadth increase in size
5	Adult in size and shape

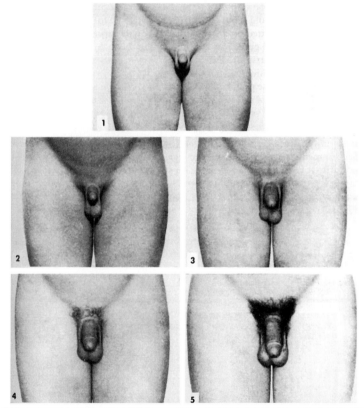

*From Seidel HM, Ball JW, Dains JE, Benedict GW: **Mosby's Guide to Physical Examination.***
St. Louis: Mosby, 1987:77.

TANNER STAGING OF MALE PUBIC HAIR DEVELOPMENT

STAGE	DESCRIPTION
1	No pubic hair; preadolescent
2	Scant, long, slightly pigmented
3	Darker, starting to curl, small amount
4	Resembles adult, but less quantity; coarse, curly
5	Adult distribution, spread to medial surface of thighs

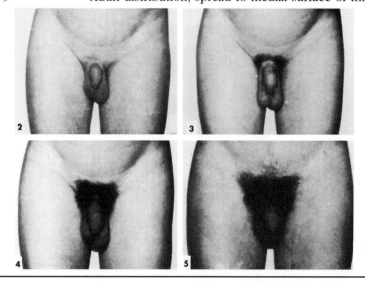

From Seidel HM, Ball JW, Dains JE, Benedict GW: Mosby's Guide to Physical Examination.
St. Louis: Mosby, 1987:76.

SEAPI STAGING SYSTEM OF URINARY INCONTINENCE

SUBJECTIVE

Stress-related leakage	0 = No urine loss
	1 = Loss with strenuous activity
	2 = Loss with moderate activity
	3 = Loss with minimal activity, or gravitational incontinence
Emptying ability	0 = No obstructive symptoms
	1 = Minimal symptoms
	2 = Significant symptoms
	3 = Voiding only in dribbles or retention
Anatomy	0 = No descent during strain
	1 = Descent, not through introitus
	2 = Descent through introitus with strain
	3 = Through introitus without strain
Protection	0 = Never used
	1 = Used only for certain occasions
	2 = Used daily for occasional accidents
	3 = Used continually for frequent accidents or constant leaking
Inhibition	0 = No urgency incontinence
	1 = Rare urgency incontinence
	2 = Urgency incontinence once per week
	3 = Urgency incontinence at least once a day

OBJECTIVE

Stress-related leakage	Observe for leak during Valsalva and cough
	0 = No leak
	1 = Leak at >80 cm water
	2 = Leak at 30–80 cm water
	3 = Leak at <30 cm water
Emptying ability	Postvoid residual should be verified by repeat measurements
	0 = 0–60 mL
	1 = 61–100 mL
	2 = 101–200 mL
	3 = >200 mL or unable to void
Anatomy	Position of bladder neck relative to symphysis during cough or Valsalva seen on lateral cystogram
	0 = Above symphysis with strain
	1 = <2 cm below symphysis with strain
	2 = >2 cm below symphysis with strain
	3 = >2 cm below symphysis at rest
Protection	0 = Never used
	1 = Used only for certain occasions
	2 = Used daily for occasional accidents
	3 = Used continually for frequent accidents or constant leaking

Table continued on following page

SEAPI STAGING SYSTEM OF URINARY INCONTINENCE *Continued*

Inhibition	Involuntary rise in pressure during cystometry
	0 = No rise in pressure
	1 = Rise late in filling (>500 mL)
	2 = Medium fill rise (150–500 mL)
	3 = Early rise (<150 mL)

A subjective (S 0 to 15) and objective (O 0 to 15) score can be assigned to each patient.

From Raz S, Eriksen D: SEAPI incontince classification system. Neurourol Urodyn 1992; 11:187.

CLASSIFICATION OF HYPOSPADIAS

Hypospadias can be classified based on the anatomic location of the meatus: glanular, distal penile, mid penile, peno-scrotal junction, scrotal, and perineal. A newer system proposed by Barcat involves straightening the penis and then describing the location of the meatus as either anterior, middle, or posterior.

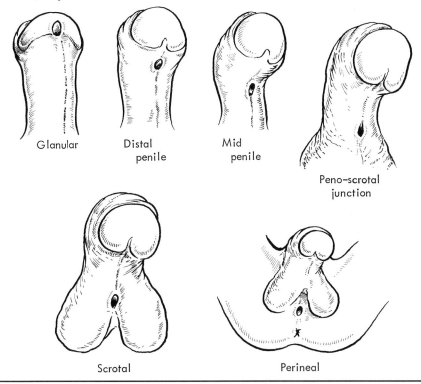

Glanular Distal penile Mid penile Peno–scrotal junction

Scrotal Perineal

From Mustardé J (ed): Plastic Surgery in Infancy and Childhood. *Philadelphia: W.B. Saunders, 1971:400.*

CHAPTER TWELVE

Neurosurgery

GRADING OF REFLEXES

GRADE	DESCRIPTION
0	Absent reflex
1	Present but diminished reflex
2	Normal reflex
3	Increased reflex
4	Markedly increased reflex

In describing reflexes, one also should designate whether the reflex required augmentation during the testing. "Aug." after the reflex score is commonly used.

From Youmans JR: Neurological Surgery, 4th ed. Philadelphia: W.B. Saunders, 1996:33.

GLASGOW OUTCOME SCALE

SCORE	DESCRIPTION	OUTCOME
5	Good recovery	Normal or near normal recovery
4	Moderate disability	Disabled but independent
3	Severe disability	Dependent with physical or psychological disabilities, or both
2	Persistent vegetative state	
1	Dead	

Although widely used, this scale is rather subjective and does not address specific aspects of neurologic recovery. Some patients who achieve a good recovery may have persisting deficits in one or more tested areas.

From Youmans JR: Neurological Surgery, 4th ed. Philadelphia: W.B. Saunders, 1996:1622.

RANCHO LOS AMIGOS HOSPITAL LEVELS OF COGNITIVE FUNCTION

LEVEL	RESPONSE
I	No response
II	Generalized response
III	Localized response
IV	Confused—agitated
V	Confused—inappropriate
VI	Confused—appropriate
VII	Automatic—appropriate
VIII	Purposeful—appropriate

From Wilkins RH, Rengachary SS (eds): **Neurosurgery, 2nd ed.** *New York: McGraw-Hill, 1996:448. Copyright 1996, The McGraw-Hill Companies, Inc.*

CLASSIFICATION OF ELECTROENCEPHALOGRAM (EEG) FREQUENCY PATTERNS

EEG FREQUENCY PATTERNS

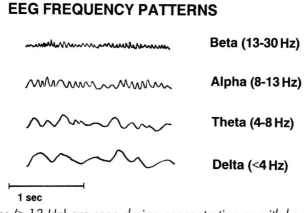

Beta (13-30 Hz)

Alpha (8-13 Hz)

Theta (4-8 Hz)

Delta (<4 Hz)

1 sec

Beta rhythms (>13 Hz) are seen during concentration or with barbiturates and benzodiazepines. Alpha rhythms (8–13 Hz) are recorded primarily over the occipital region in an alert, relaxed person whose eyes are closed. This pattern also can be seen during light anesthesia. Theta rhythms (4–8 Hz) are recorded during general anesthesia. Delta rhythms (<4 Hz) occur during deep sleep, deep anesthesia, and several pathologic states (ischemia, drug overdose, metabolic disorders).

From Kirby, Gravenstein (eds): **Clinical Anesthesia Practice.** *Philadelphia: W.B. Saunders, 1994:400.*

CLINICAL CLASSIFICATION OF CORTICAL APHASIAS

TYPE	SPEECH	REPETITION	COMPREHENSION	NAMING	SIGNS	LESIONS
Broca's	Nonfluent	Impaired	Normal	Marginally impaired	RHP, RHH apraxia of left limbs, face	Left posterior inferior frontal
Wernicke's	Fluent	Impaired	Impaired	Impaired		Left posterior superior temporal
Conduction	Fluent	Impaired	Normal	Impaired (paraphasic)	±RHS, apraxia of all limbs and face	Left parietal
Global	Nonfluent	Impaired	Impaired	Impaired	RHP, RHS, HRH	Left frontal temporal parietal
Anomic	Fluent	Normal	Normal	Impaired	None	Left posterior inferior temporal, or temporal-occipital
Transcortical motor	Nonfluent	Normal	Normal	Impaired	RHP	Left medial front or anterior border zone
Sensory	Fluent	Normal	Impaired	Impaired	±HRH	Left medial parietal or posterior border zone
Mixed	Nonfluent	Normal	Impaired	Impaired	RHP, RHS	Left medial frontal parietal or complete border zone

HRH, homonymous right hemianopsia; RHP, right hemiparesis; RHS, right hemisensory defect.

From Kandel ER, Schwartz JA, Jessell TM: Principles of Neural Science, 3rd ed. East Norwalk, CT: Appleton & Lange, 1992:847.

CLASSIFICATION OF SEVERE HEAD INJURY BY COMPUTED TOMOGRAPHY (CT) CATEGORIES

CLASSIFICATION	DESCRIPTION
Diffuse injury I (no visible pathology)	No visible intracranial pathology seen on CT
Diffuse injury II	Cisterns are present with midline shift 0–5 mm and/or lesion densities present No high- or mixed-density lesion >25 cm³ May include bone fragments and foreign bodies
Diffuse injury III (swelling)	Cisterns compressed or absent with shift 0–5 mm No high- or mixed-density lesion >25 cm³
Diffuse injury IV (shift)	Shift >5 mm No high- or mixed-density lesion >25 cm³
Evacuated mass lesion	Any surgically evacuated lesion
Nonevacuated mass lesion	High- or mixed-density lesion <25 cm³, not surgically evacuated

Marshall and colleagues introduced this grading system as a way of predicting outcome following head injury. Their data showed that 61.6% of diffuse injury I patients had a good recovery or moderate disability, 32.5% of diffuse injury II patients had such a recovery, 16.4% of diffuse injury III patients had a good recovery, and 6.2% of diffuse injury IV patients had a good recovery.

Table from Youmans JR: Neurological Surgery, 4th ed. Philadelphia: W.B. Saunders, 1996: 1800. Data from Marshall LF, Gautille T, Klauber MR, et al.: The outcome of severe closed head injury. J Neurosurg 1991; 75(suppl):S28–S36; and Marshall LF, Marshall SB, Klauber MR, et al.: The diagnosis of head injury requires a classification based on computed axial tomography. J Neurotrauma, 1992; 9(suppl 1):S287–S292.

CEREBRAL CONTUSION INDEX

DEPTH OF CONTUSION	GRADE
Absent	0
Does not extend through full thickness of cortex	1
Affects full thickness of cortex	2
Extends into white matter	3

EXTENT OF CONTUSION	GRADE
Absent	0
Localized	1
Moderately extensive	2
Extensive	3

The contusion index is derived from depth × extent and can range from 0 (contusions absent) to 3 × 3 = 9 (deep and extensive contusions). Contusions are usually more severe in patients with a skull fracture and usually more severe in the frontal and temporal lobes.

From Adams JH, Scott G, Parker LS, et al.: The contusion index: A quantitative approach to cerebral contusions in head injury. Neuropathol Appl Neurobiol 1980; 6:319–324.

GRADING OF SUBARACHNOID HEMORRHAGE

GRADE	DESCRIPTION
BOTTERELL SCALE	
1	Conscious with or without signs of blood in the subarachnoid space
2	Drowsy without significant neurological deficit
3	Drowsy with neurological deficit and probably intracerebral clot
4	Major neurological deficit and deterioration due to large intracerebral clot, or older age with less severe neurological deficit but preexisting cerebrovascular disease
5	Moribund or near-moribund with failing vital centers and extensor rigidity
HUNT AND HESS SCALE*	
1	Asymptomatic or minimal headache and slight nuchal rigidity
2	Moderate to severe headache, nuchal rigidity, no neurological deficit other than cranial nerve palsy
3	Drowsiness, confusion, or mild focal deficit
4	Stupor, moderate to severe hemiparesis, possible early decerebrate rigidity, and vegetative disturbances
5	Deep coma, decerebrate rigidity, moribund appearance
WORLD FEDERATION OF NEUROLOGICAL SURGEONS SCALE	
1	Glasgow coma score 15, no motor deficit
2	Glasgow coma score 13 to 14, no motor deficit
3	Glasgow coma score 13 to 14, with motor deficit
4	Glasgow coma score 7 to 12, with or without motor deficit
5	Glasgow coma score 3 to 6, with or without motor deficit

* Patients are moved into the next worst category if they have vasospasm on angiography or serious systemic disease, such as hypertension, diabetes, atherosclerosis, or chronic lung disease.

From **Youmans JR: Neurological Surgery, 4th ed. Philadelphia: W.B. Saunders, 1996:1234.**

COMPUTED TOMOGRAPHY (CT) CLASSIFICATION OF THALAMIC HEMORRHAGE

CLASS	CRITERIA
Ia	Localized in thalamus without V
Ib	Localized in thalamus with V
IIa	Extends to internal capsule without V
IIb	Extends to internal capsule with V
IIIa	Extends to hypothalamus or midbrain without V
IIIb	Extends to hypothalamus or midbrain with V

V, massive ventricular hemorrhage.

From **Wilkins RH, Rengachary SS (eds): Neurosurgery, 2nd ed. New York: McGraw-Hill, 1996:2571. Copyright 1996, The McGraw-Hill Companies, Inc.**

FISHER GRADING OF SUBARACHNOID HEMORRHAGE
▷ Using Computed Tomography (CT) Data

GRADE	DESCRIPTION	VASOSPASM RISK
1	No detectable blood on CT scan	Low
2	Diffuse blood that does not appear dense enough to represent a large, thick homogeneous clot	Low
3	Dense collection of blood that appears to represent a clot more than 1 mm thick in the vertical plane (interhemispheric fissure, insular cistern, or ambient cistern) or greater than 5 × 3 mm in longitudinal and transverse dimension in horizontal plane (stem of sylvian fissure, sylvian cistern, interpeduncular cistern)	High
4	Intracerebral or intraventricular clots but with only diffuse blood or no blood in basal cisterns	Low

Modified from Fisher CM, Kistler JP, Davis JM: Relation of cerebral vasospasm to subarachnoid hemorrhage visualized by computerized tomographic scanning. Neurosurgery 1980; 6:1.

COMPUTED TOMOGRAPHY (CT) CLASSIFICATION OF BASAL GANGLIONIC HEMORRHAGE

CLASS	TYPE	CRITERIA
I	External capsule	Localized at outside of internal capsule
II	Capsular	Extends to anterior limb of internal capsule
IIIa	Cp without V	Extends to anterior limb of internal capsule
IIIb	Cp with V	
IVa	Ca + p without V	Extends to anterior and posterior limbs of internal capsule
IVb	Ca + p with V Th	
V		Extends to thalamus or subthalamus

a, anterior; C, capsule; p, posterior; Th, thalamus; V, massive ventricular hemorrhage.

From Wilkins RH, Rengachary SS (eds): Neurosurgery, 2nd ed. New York: McGraw-Hill, 1996:2571. Copyright 1996, The McGraw-Hill Companies, Inc.

CLASSIFICATION OF INTRACRANIAL ARTERIAL ANEURYSMS

I. MORPHOLOGY
   A. Saccular
   B. Fusiform
   C. Dissecting
   D. Microaneurysm (Charcot-Bouchard)
II. SIZE
   A. <3 mm
   B. 4-6 mm (small)
   C. 7-10 mm (medium)
   D. 11-25 mm (large)
   E. >25 mm (giant)
III. LOCATION
   A. Anterior circulation arteries
      1. Internal carotid
         a. Carotid canal
         b. Intracavernous
         c. Paraclinoid (ophthalmic)
         d. Posterior communicating region
         e. Anterior choroidal region
         f. Carotid bifurcation
      2. Anterior cerebral
         a. A1 (main branch)
         b. Anterior communicating region
         c. A2 (distal): callosomarginal region or distal pericallosal
      3. Middle cerebral
         a. M1 (main branch): lenticulostriate or temporal branch regions
         b. Bifurcation
         c. Peripheral
   B. Posterior circulation arteries
      1. Vertebral
         a. Main trunk
         b. Posterior inferior cerebellar artery region
      2. Basilar
         a. Bifurcation
         b. Superior cerebellar artery region
         c. Anterior inferior cerebellar artery region
         d. Basilar trunk
         e. Vertebrobasilar junction region
      3. Posterior cerebral
         a. P1 (first branches of basilar—distal to apex)
         b. P2 (distal posterior cerebral)

From Wilkins RH, Rengachary SS (eds): Neurosurgery, 2nd ed. New York: McGraw-Hill, 1996:1309. Copyright 1996, The McGraw-Hill Companies, Inc.

CLASSIFICATION OF CHIARI MALFORMATIONS

TYPE	DESCRIPTION
I	Elongation of the cerebellar tonsils into conical extensions that accompany the medulla into the cervical canal
II	Downward displacement of the vermis, 4th ventricle, and lower brain stem, into the spinal canal
III	Displacement of nearly the entire cerebellum as well as the 4th ventricle into the cervical canal
IV	Cerebellar hypoplasia (not a true hernia)

From Youmans JR: **Neurological Surgery, 4th ed. Philadelphia: W.B. Saunders, 1996:1090.**

CLASSIFICATION OF NEUROFIBROMATOSIS

TYPE 1
A diagnosis is established if any two of the following features exist:
1. Six café au lait macules more than 5 mm in greatest diameter if prepubertal, or more than 15 mm if postpubertal
2. Two or more neurofibromas of any type, or one plexiform neurofibroma
3. Axillary or inguinal freckling
4. A distinctive osseous lesion, such as sphenoid dysplasia, congenital bowing, or thinning of long bone cortex, with or without pseudoarthrosis
5. Bilateral optic nerve gliomas
6. Two or more iris Lisch nodules
7. A first-degree relative with neurofibromatosis Type 1, diagnosed by the above criteria

TYPE 2
1. Bilateral vestibular schwannomas demonstrated by computed tomography or magnetic resonance imaging
   OR
2. A first-degree relative with bilateral vestibular schwannomas and either a unilateral vestibular schwannoma or any two of the following: neurofibroma, meningioma, glioma, schwannoma, posterior lens opacity

From Youmans JR: **Neurological Surgery, 4th ed. Philadelphia: W.B. Saunders, 1996:818.**

CLASSIFICATION OF HYDROCEPHALUS

NONCOMMUNICATING

I. Congenital lesions
A. Aqueductal obstruction (stenosis)
1. Gliosis
2. Fording
3. True narrowing
4. Septum
B. Atresia of the foramina of Luschka and Magendie (Dandy-Walker cyst)
C. Masses
1. Benign intracranial cysts
2. Vascular malformation
3. Tumors

II. Acquired lesions
A. Aqueductal stenosis (gliosis)
B. Ventricular inflammations and scars
C. Masses
1. Tumors
2. Non-neoplastic masses

COMMUNICATING

I. Congenital lesions
A. Arnold-Chiari malformation
B. Encephalocele
C. Leptomeningeal inflammations
D. Lissencephaly
E. Congenital absence of arachnoidal granulations

II. Acquired lesions
A. Leptomeningeal inflammations
1. Infections
2. Hemorrhage
3. Particulate matter
B. Masses
1. Tumors
2. Non-neoplastic masses
C. Platybasia

III. Oversecretion of cerebrospinal fluid (choroid plexus papilloma)

From Wilkins RH, Rengachary SS (eds): Neurosurgery, 2nd ed. New York: McGraw-Hill, 1996:3626. Copyright 1996, The McGraw-Hill Companies, Inc.

GRADING OF ASTROCYTIC TUMORS

WHO DESIGNATION	WHO GRADE	KERNOHAN GRADE	ST. ANNE-MAYO GRADE	ST. ANNE-MAYO CRITERIA
Pilocytic astrocytoma	I	I	Excluded	No criteria fulfilled
Astrocytoma	II	I, II	1	One criterion: usually nuclear atypia
			2	Two criteria: usually nuclear atypia and mitosis
Anaplastic (malignant) astrocytoma	III	II, III	3	
Glioblastoma	IV	III, IV	4	Three or four criteria: usually the above and endothelial proliferation and/or necrosis

All of these grading systems impart a worse prognosis as the grade increases. The future trend is toward molecular analysis of tumor cells, with grading based on genetic studies.

WHO, World Health Organization.

From Youmans JR: Neurological Surgery, 4th ed. Philadelphia: W.B. Saunders, 1996:2644.

WORLD HEALTH ORGANIZATION (WHO) CLASSIFICATION OF TUMORS OF THE MENINGES (1993)

I. TUMORS OF MENINGOTHELIAL CELLS
A. Meningioma
1. Meningothelial
2. Fibrous (fibroblastic)
3. Transitional (mixed)
4. Psammomatous
5. Angiomatous
6. Microcystic
7. Secretory
8. Clear cell
9. Choroid
10. Lymphoplasmacyte-rich
11. Metaplastic
B. Atypical meningioma
C. Papillary meningioma
D. Anaplastic (malignant) meningioma

II. MESENCHYMAL, NONMENINGOTHELIAL TUMORS
A. Benign neoplasms
1. Osteocartilaginous tumors
2. Lipoma
3. Fibrous histiocytoma
4. Others
B. Malignant neoplasms
1. Hemangiopericytoma
2. Chondrosarcoma
Variant: mesenchymal chondrosarcoma
3. Malignant fibrous histiocytoma
4. Rhabdomyosarcoma
5. Meningeal sarcomatosis
6. Others
C. Primary melanocytic lesions
1. Diffuse melanosis
2. Melanocytoma
3. Malignant melanoma
Variant: meningeal melanomatosis
D. Tumors of uncertain histogenesis
1. Hemangioblastoma
(capillary hemangioblastoma)

From Wilkins RH, Rengachary SS (eds): Neurosurgery, 2nd ed. New York: McGraw-Hill, 1996:845. Copyright 1996, The McGraw-Hill Companies, Inc.

SIMPSON GRADE OF INTRACRANIAL TUMOR REMOVAL

GRADE	DESCRIPTION
I	Macroscopically complete tumor removal with excision of the tumor's dural attachment and any abnormal bone
II	Macroscopically complete tumor removal with coagulation of its dural attachment
III	Macroscopically complete removal of the intradural tumor without resection or coagulation of its dural attachment or extradural extensions
IV	Subtotal removal of the tumor
V	Simple decompression of tumor

From Simpson D: The recurrence of intracranial meningiomas after surgical treatment. J Neurol Neurosurg Psychiatry 1957; 20:22–39.

CLASSIFICATION OF PITUITARY TUMORS

RADIOLOGIC	ANATOMIC		SURGICAL
A. Sella Turcica			
Grade 0:	Intact, normal contour		
Grade I:	Intact, focal bulging	Micro	Enclosed
Grade II:	Intact, enlarged	Macro	
Grade III:	Destroyed, partially		Invasive
Grade IV:	Destroyed, totally		
Grade V:	Distant spread via cerebrospinal fluid or blood		
B. Extrasellar Extensions			
Suprasellar			
A.	Suprasellar cistern		
B.	Recesses third ventricle		
C.	Whole anterior third ventricle		
Parasellar	(Asymmetrical)		
D.	Intracranial intradural		
	Anterior		
	Midline		
	Posterior		
E.	Extracranial extradural (lateral cavernous)		

From Wilkins RH, Rengachary SS (eds): Neurosurgery, 2nd ed. New York: McGraw-Hill, 1996:1376. Copyright 1996, The McGraw-Hill Companies, Inc.

CLASSIFICATION OF CEREBRAL EDEMA BASED ON PATHOGENESIS

TYPE	PATHOGENESIS	COMPOSITION	LOCATION	CEREBROSPINAL FLUID FORMATION RATE	BLOOD-BRAIN BARRIER (BBB)
Vasogenic	BBB breakdown	Water, Na+, and plasma proteins	Primary extracellular, secondary intracellular	Not increased	Disturbed
Cytoxic	Disturbance of cellular metabolism	Water, Na+	Intracellular		Undisturbed
Osmotic	Osmotic gradient	Water	Intracellular extracellular	Increased	Undisturbed
Hydrostatic	Hydrostatic gradient	Water, Na+	Extracellular		Undisturbed

From Wilkins RH, Rengachary SS (eds): Neurosurgery, 2nd ed. New York: McGraw-Hill, 1996:341. Copyright 1996, The McGraw-Hill Companies, Inc.

FUNCTIONAL LEVELS IN QUADRAPLEGIA

LEVEL	FUNCTION PRESENT	MUSCLES FUNCTIONING
C5	Shoulder abduction	Deltoid
	Elbow flexion	Biceps
C6	Wrist extension	Brachioradialis
		Extensor carpi
		Radialis longus and brevis
		Pronator teres
C7	Elbow extension	Triceps
	Finger extension	Extensor digitorum communis
	Wrist flexion	Flexor carpi radialis
C8	Finger flexion	Flexor digitorum profundus
T1	Intrinsic hand muscle function	Intrinsic hand muscles

From Wilkins RH, Rengachary SS (eds): Neurosurgery, 2nd ed. New York: McGraw-Hill, 1996:453. Copyright 1996, The McGraw-Hill Companies, Inc.

CHAPTER THIRTEEN

Anesthesia

NEW YORK HEART ASSOCIATION FUNCTIONAL CLASSIFICATION

CLASS	DESCRIPTION
I	Patients with cardiac disease but without resulting limitations of physical activity. Ordinary physical activity does not cause undue fatigue, palpitation, dyspnea, or anginal pain.
II	Patients with cardiac disease resulting in slight limitation of physical activity. They are comfortable at rest. Ordinary physical activity results in fatigue, palpitation, dyspnea, or anginal pain.
III	Patients with cardiac disease resulting in marked limitation of physical activity. They are comfortable at rest. Less than ordinary physical activity causes fatigue, palpitation, dyspnea, or anginal pain.
IV	Patients with cardiac disease resulting in inability to carry on any physical activity without discomfort. Symptoms of cardiac insufficiency or of the anginal syndrome may be present even at rest. If any physical activity is undertaken, discomfort is increased.

From American Heart Association: New York Heart Association functional classification. In Braunwald E. (ed): Heart Disease, 2nd ed. Philadelphia: W.B. Saunders, 1984.

AMERICAN SOCIETY OF ANESTHESIOLOGY STANDARDS FOR BASIC INTRAOPERATIVE MONITORING

STANDARD	DESCRIPTION
I	Qualified anesthesia personnel shall be present in the room throughout the conduct of all general anesthetics, regional anesthetics, and monitored anesthesia care.
II	During all anesthetics, the patient's oxygenation, ventilation, circulation, and temperature shall be continually evaluated.

From Longnecker DE, Tinker JH, Morgan GE: Principles and Practice of Anesthesiology, 2nd ed. St. Louis: Mosby, 1998:2626.

CLASSIFICATION OF AIRWAYS

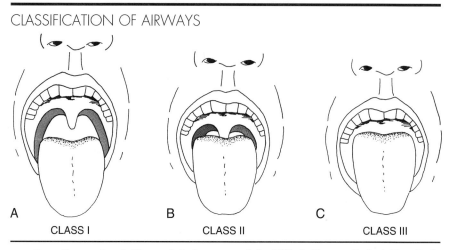

A	B	C
CLASS I	CLASS II	CLASS III

From Ovassapian A: **Fiberoptic Endoscopy and the Difficult Airway, 2nd ed. New York: Lippincott-Raven, 1996.**

GOLDMAN CARDIAC RISK INDEX

VARIABLE	POINT VALUE
Third heart sound or jugular venous distention	11
Recent myocardial infarction	10
Nonsinus rhythm or premature atrial contractions	7
More than 5 premature ventricular contractions	7
Age more than 70 years	5
Emergency operation	4
Poor general medical condition	3
Intraperitoneal, intrathoracic, or aortic operation	3
Important valvular aortic stenosis	3

Add point values together and determine Goldman class.

CLASS	POINT RANGE	% CARDIAC COMPLICATION
I	0–5	1
II	6–12	7
III	13–25	14
IV	>26	78

The Goldman CRI predicts the risk of a cardiac complication associated with a noncardiac procedure.

From Goldman L, Caldera DL, Nussbaum SR, et al.: **Multifactorial index of cardiac risk in noncardiac surgical procedures. N Engl J Med 1977; 297:845.**

CLASSIFICATION OF LOCAL ANESTHETICS

GROUP I—BENZOIC ACID ESTERS
Benzocaine
Butacaine
Chlorprocaine
Cyclomethycaine
Isobucaine
Meprylcaine
Metabutethamine
Piperocaine
Procaine
Tetracaine

GROUP II—AMIDES (OTHERS)
Bupivacaine
Dibucaine
Dicyclomine
Lidocaine
Mepivacaine
Oxethazaine
Phenacaine

Group I anesthetics cross-react with each other, but not with amides. The group II drugs do not cross-react with each other.

From Longnecker DE, Tinker JH, Morgan GE: **Principles and Practice of Anesthesiology,** *2nd ed. St. Louis: Mosby, 1998:2397.*

AMERICAN SOCIETY OF ANESTHESIOLOGY (ASA) PHYSICAL STATUS CLASSIFICATION

ASA CLASS	DESCRIPTION
I	No Organic Disease
II	Mild or moderate systemic disease without functional impairment
III	Organic disease with definite functional impairment
IV	Severe disease that is life threatening
V	Moribund patient, not expected to survive without surgery
VI	Brain-dead organ donor

From Longnecker DE, Tinker JH, Morgan GE: **Principles and Practice of Anesthesiology,** *2nd ed. St. Louis: Mosby, 1998.*

INDEX

Note: Page numbers in *italics* refer to illustrations.